BELOW THE BELT

A guide to gynaecological problems

Vivienne Welburn

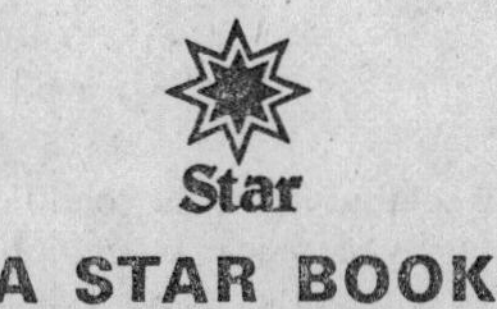

A STAR BOOK

published by
the Paperback Division of
W. H. ALLEN & Co. Ltd

A Star Book
Published in 1982
by the Paperback Division of
W.H. Allen & Co. Ltd
A Howard and Wyndham Company
44 Hill Street, London W1X 8LB

Typeset by V & M Graphics Ltd., Aylesbury, Bucks.

Printed in Great Britain by
Hun ı Barnard Printing Ltd., Aylesbury, Bucks.

ISBN 0 352 306858

BELOW THE BELT

A Star Original

Vivienne Welburn was born in Yorkshire in 1941. After graduating from Leeds University she taught English in London comprehensive schools for eight years whilst writing for the theatre.

Her first professional production was at the Traverse Theatre Club in Edinburgh in 1965. Her published plays are *Johnny So Long* and *The Drag* (1967); *Clear Way* (1967); *The Treadwheel* and *Coil Without Dreams* (1975). She also contributed to *Play Ten*, a book of short plays for schools (1977). She has since branched out into journalism and book writing. Her book *Postnatal Depression* was published by Fontana in 1980.

Vivienne Welburn currently works as a freelance writer. She lives in Chiswick with her two daughters Imogen and Pippa.

Contents

Preface

This book owes its existence to the fact that in 1971 a group of women in Boston produced a book which revolutionised attitudes to women's health care. *Our Bodies Ourselves* was the first health book written by women for women. It approached health as something embracing the whole of life and worked from the experiences of women outwards to the 'objective' facts of medical science. It critically examined the structure of the health care system and noted the ways it failed to meet women's needs.

There have been many books since dealing in more or less detail with different aspects of women's health. I am pleased to include this one amongst their number. I have chosen to limit its scope to the area of greatest embarrassment, the area below the belt which contains our sexual, reproductive and genito-urinary organs.

My approach has been to talk first to women about the problems which they experience both with their bodies and their doctors and then to talk to doctors and consult their books. The result is a handbook of information which I hope will be useful to women.

I must thank first all the women who talked to me so openly about their medical histories. My gratitude is also due to the many doctors who gave up their time to talk to me and explain things from their point of view. Above all my thanks to my husband and children for their patience and support during the months in which I was locked in my study writing.

Chapter One

Genital Geography

Men and women have different bodies, that we can agree. Nothing wrong with that, *vive la difference* and so on. However, for most of us as women, it is our bodies and the fact that they *are* different that gives us so many of the problems that we have to deal with in life, both social, emotional and physical.

The sad fact is that the male body has always been taken as the norm from which female bodies differ. They have problems, we have 'special' problems. Indeed, we are persuaded to see the normal functions of menstruation, pregnancy, birth and menopause as problems in themselves, deviations, forms of weakness which make us unsuitable for an active rôle in the world.

But whilst our bodily functions are hushed up and hidden by medical mystique and social taboo, our bodily form is everywhere displayed for consumption. It is impossible to escape from the bombardment of images of the stereotyped Desirable Woman. The stereotype was described by Germaine Greer over a decade ago:

> The gynolatry of our civilisation is written large upon its face, upon hoardings, cinema screens, television, newspapers, magazines, tins, packets, cartons, bottles, all consecrated to the reigning deity, the female fetish. Her dominion must not be thought to entail the rule of women, for she is not a woman ... Her essential quality is castratedness. She absolutely must be young, her body hairless, her flesh buoyant, and *she must not have a sexual organ.**

**The Female Eunuch*, Germaine Greer, Paladin 1971.

She is with us still, this female who is all form and no content. She does not have periods, let alone period pains, nor pregnancies, wanted or otherwise. She does not suffer from cystitis or thrush; she is never overweight; her breasts don't sag. She is as deodorised, perfumed and plastic as she ever was and we are coaxed into accepting her as our model.

So, to a great extent, are doctors, who should know better but often choose not to. They do, after all, share the same culture and suffer from the same illusions of what represents a 'real' woman and her functions. Indeed, it has been argued that medicine acts as a method of socially controlling women by proving 'scientifically' that our normal functions are 'sick', our mental health precarious and our behaviour irrational.

Be that as it may, it is certainly the experience of women that when they are afflicted with female complaints they receive scant attention and are given virtually no information:

> The doctor told me nothing. I'd like to have known something. You know, if I've got something, I'd rather know what it is I've got and a bit about it.

This was a very typical response from most of the women I interviewed for this book, whether they were suffering from menstrual problems, vaginal infections or any other gynaecological troubles. But more of that in the next chapter.

It was inevitable, given the problems and contradictions we face over our biology, that the desire to understand and gain some control over our bodies would become vital. So it happened that women decided to learn the language and secrets of doctors in order to make their own assessment of what ailed them.

Knowledge is information and there is nothing magical about medical information. It is unlikely that any of us would wish to know as much as the average doctor or to dispense with doctors altogether. But a working knowledge of your own body not only helps to dispel many fears, it also enables you to ask the right questions of your doctor and to go on asking until you receive a satisfactory answer.

Body image

The saying that inside every fat person is a thin person trying to get out demonstrates the truth that we do not necessarily see ourselves as others see us. Some very pretty women are convinced they are unattractive, some rather plain women can convince us of their beauty. Most women seem to believe there is *something* wrong with them, which is what keeps plastic surgeons in business.

Our first relationship as babies is with our bodies and the simple, physical need for food, sleep and touch. At that age those needs are our very lives and we are all body. It is only later that we come to distinguish between ourselves and others and later still that we separate our thinking, feeling selves from our physical form, our bodies.

The separation is, of course, totally artificial and can be damaging in the effect it has on our sexuality and our health. It is not an easy division to overcome but a start can be made by seeing, touching and smelling our own bodies, becoming familiar with and accepting the reality of what we have and are.

It is only by knowing and feeling comfortable with the body that we have that we can hope to combat the effect of the stereotypes that we have to cope with. We know that society attributes certain qualities to different body shapes: slim is sexy, fat is jolly, tall is graceful or Amazonian, depending on build, short is fragile. If you are slim and small busted you will be 'boyish' and if plump and large busted you will be 'voluptuous'. The stereotype may fit comfortably but if it doesn't it may be necessary to change your own image of your body and see yourself in a new light.

Remember that it is important to see and examine the whole of your body in detail. Here I shall concentrate on the body below the belt. If you feel ready to examine yourself begin by making yourself comfortable in a room with good lighting, a long mirror, a hand mirror and a lock on the door. If you have not examined yourself before it may be a moment of truth to discover how acutely embarrassed you feel. Most women do. The feeling wears off with practice and familiarity, luckily, so persevere.

Strip off from the waist down (or, better still, strip completely if the room is warm enough) and stand in front of a full-length mirror. What you see is your body, it's you, it's important, it matters. Look carefully and then caress your body. Stroke the stomach, round the buttocks, down the thighs, up the inside thigh and back over the stomach. You probably feel rather silly, but it is much easier to learn to know and like your body if you enjoy touching it.

Body hair

The most immediately noticeable area is the pubic hair. There was a time when pubic hair was considered rude and nude pin-ups had it carefully painted out. It was considered rude because body hair represents animal sexuality and animal sexuality was very much not approved of.

Attitudes are now much more liberal. But women still find it necessary to remove hair from their legs and armpits, at least British and American women do. French and Italian women don't seem to worry so much. It goes without saying, of course, that body hair is entirely natural. It's supposed to be there and a lot of men like it to be there.

In fact body hair does have a function. There are tiny scent glands based in the pubic and armpit areas. When the female is sexually aroused these glands send off a scent which is attractive to the male. The hair traps this smell and prevents it from evaporating. The very word 'smell' is enough to send most women off to grab a flannel and deodorant, which is a great pity because, as a rule, it is only stale body odour which is offensive.

Pubic hair is coarse and crinkly. You may have a great deal or very little; it may reach down your thighs or grow up towards your navel. No two women are the same and it is not especially helpful to think in terms of average or normal hair growth.

If you stroke your body from your navel down to your pubic hair, you will notice that where the triangle of pubic hair starts, there is a bump. This is fatty tissue which covers the joint of the pubic bones which are part of the pelvic bones or hip girdle. This bump is called the *mons veneris* (most medical terms are Latin – this one means mountain of Venus, for obvious reasons). If you press down on the bump you will easily be able to feel the bone underneath.

That's about all that you can see of your genitals when you're standing up and, sadly, that's all that thousands of women have ever seen of them since mothers in the past have generally pursued a 'hands off' policy with their daughters. The next stage, therefore, is to sit or squat and use a hand mirror to see what you actually possess in that hidden area between your legs. Again, remember that the more often you do this, the less embarrassing it becomes.

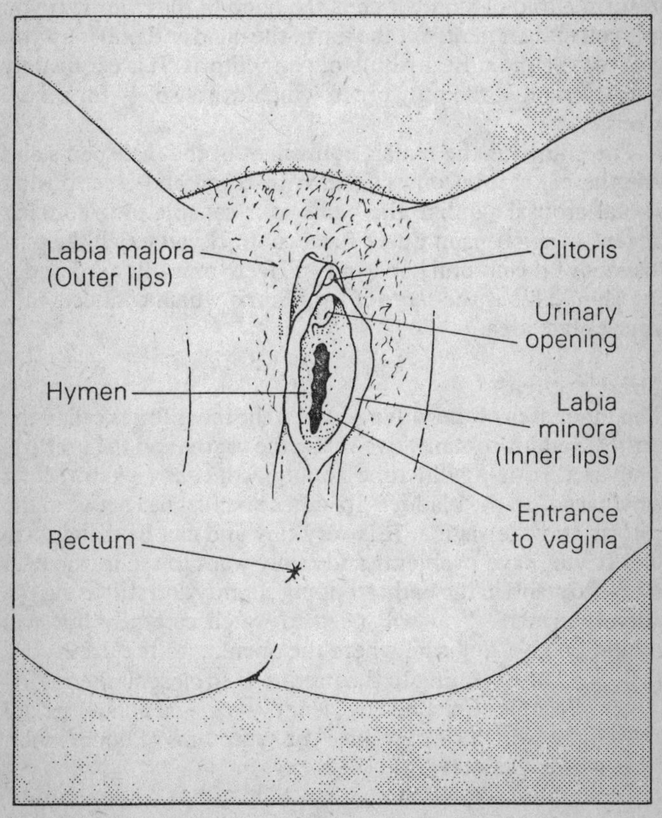

The vulva

The genital area which you can see when you look in the hand mirror is called the vulva. There are, as you will see, two sets of lips or *labia* which protect the very sensitive inner areas and keep them moist. The outer lips (labia majora) are thick and fatty and covered with pubic hair. The inner lips (labia minora) are long, hairless folds of skin. They vary in size from woman to woman and may reach out beyond the outer lips. In colour they may be anything from light pink to dark brown and in texture may be smooth or wrinkled.

The inner lips join together at the top just below the mons to form a fold of skin which is the hood of the *clitoris*. If you put your finger gently at the top of the hood and pull it up you will see the pink, fleshy bulb of your clitoris. It is exquisitely sensitive and is the only organ which exists solely for sexual arousal.

The clitoris is the female equivalent of the male penis and like the penis it becomes filled with blood and erect during sexual arousal. Unlike the penis, it is capable of producing dozens of orgasms in quick succession. If you touch the part just above the clitoral hood you will feel a movable cord under the skin. This is the *shaft* of the clitoris which connects into your pelvic area.

The Urethra

The inner area of the vulva between the inner lips is called the *vestibule* and it contains two holes, the vagina and the urethra. The urethra is a thin tube about 1½ inches (3.5 cm) long which leads to the bladder. Its outer opening lies between the clitoris and the vagina. It is very tiny and can be difficult to see. If you have problems and really want to see it, the best idea is to stand in the bath, stooping slightly and still using the mirror, urinate. You will need to watch carefully but you should be able to locate where the opening to the urethra is.

Because the opening to the urethra is so close to the vagina it can become irritated by lengthy or strenuous sexual intercourse which can produce the symptoms of honeymoon cystitis (see Chapter 5).

The Vagina

The opening to the vagina is the larger and more obvious of the two holes within the vestibule. If you are a virgin, you may be able to see the *hymen*. It is a thin strip of membrane which lies across the lower part of the vaginal opening. Occasionally it may cover the opening completely which can cause problems, especially if it is also very tough. One woman told me:

> My hymen was virtually like a built-in chastity belt, it was unbreakable except by operation. I was never able to use a tampon. Everybody used to say, 'Of course you can, don't be silly,' and I said, 'I haven't got a hole there,' and they said, 'Everybody has a hole there.' But I had no hole. Anyway, at the age of twenty I got a tampon stuck inside me and I couldn't get it out. I was in the States at the time. I had surgical removal. I suppose it was the best way of finding out there was something wrong.

This is, needless to say, a rare occurrence, but it does show the value of self examination. Usually the hymen can be stretched before intercourse by using a tampon or by simply stretching it gently with your fingers. The absence of an intact hymen is no proof that you have experienced sex, nor is the presence of one necessarily proof of virginity. In fact all women still have a hymen and if yours has been stretched you may notice the irregular tissue stretching across the lower part of your vagina.

The vagina itself is amazingly soft and elastic. It is a muscular tube which connects the womb to the outside of the body. The word itself comes from the Latin and means 'sheath'; doctors call it the 'front passage'. When the vagina is empty its walls touch each other and there is no space there at all, rather like a glove. It is composed of folds of skin which stretch to mould themselves around whatever is inserted whether it is a tampon, fingers or a penis. Usually the vagina is about 4 inches (9 cm) long and about 1 inch in diameter but during sexual arousal it can extend an additional 2 inches (5 cm) in length and an extra inch in diameter. It can dilate much further than that, of course, to allow the passage of a baby during birth.

First make sure that your hands are clean and then insert two fingers into your vagina and you will feel the soft folds. It may be easier for you to examine yourself if you stand with one foot on a small stool. You may find that you are fairly dry inside or very wet, depending on what stage of the menstrual cycle you are in. During sexual arousal vaginal secretions increase considerably and these secretions, which taste rather salty, are continuous during the fertile years. They serve the purpose of both providing lubrication and helping to keep the vagina clean and acid. The acidic state of the vagina is important because it helps to kill off any invading germs.

In childhood and after the menopause there are fewer secretions. This rarely causes problems for children but it can make intercourse difficult and painful for older women as well as providing them with less protection against infection. The mouth of the vagina is very sensitive and rich in nerve endings but the rest of the vagina has very little feeling. The inside of the vagina is sealed off at the top by the cervix. This makes it impossible to lose a tampon or anything else up into the body. Anything inserted in the vagina will stay there until it is removed.

If you press gently on the roof of the vagina you will notice that you have an urge to urinate. This is because the bottom of the bladder lies just above the top of the vagina and is separated from it by very thin tissue. The bottom of the vagina is similarly separated from the top of the rectum or back passage.

Whilst you still have your fingers in your vagina, try tensing the vagina muscles. It is easiest to do this by pretending that you are stopping a flow of urine mid-stream. Slowly tense the muscles as tightly as you can and then slowly relax them. By doing this you are contracting the muscles of your pelvic floor. These muscles are very important and if they sag you may have problems controlling your urine. Sometimes this can lead to a prolapse if the womb sags down into the vagina (see Chapter 10).

You can strengthen your pelvic floor muscles in the same

way you strengthen other muscles, by exercise. The easy thing about exercising these muscles is that you can do it at any time, anywhere. Simply tighten the muscles as hard as you can, hold it for a count of three and gently relax. Do this about ten times for each exercise and then build it up to more. This is described in fuller detail in Chapter 10.

There are two pea-sized glands which lie one on each side of the opening to the vagina. These are called Bartholin's glands. They produce a thin mucus which helps to lubricate the vulva and vagina. It is useful to know about them because sometimes they get infected and swell when they can be extremely painful.

If you look once more at your genital area, you will see an area of skin between the inner lips of the vulva and the anus. This is called the *perineum*. If you touch it you will find that it is very sensitive. This is the place which is so often cut during birth, but more of that later (see Chapter 12). The anus is the entrance to the back passage or rectum which is the last part of the large intestine.

The cervix

To feel your cervix you might find it easier to squat, but if you prefer to stand with one foot on a stool it will be helpful to bend forward slightly. You will notice that as you move your fingers into your vagina they slide at an angle towards the small of your back, not straight upwards.

The cervix is a fleshy knob which has a firm, smooth, rubbery surface, rather like the tip of the nose. There is what feels like a small dimple at the centre which is called the *os*. This is the opening to the cervical (serve-eye-ical) canal which leads to the uterus or womb. The os is about as wide as a very thin straw, or, if you have had a baby, it will be a horizontal slit about ¼ of an inch long. It is so small it is impossible for a finger, tampon or penis to go through it. It is, however, capable of stretching to allow a baby through during birth.

The cervix is sensitive to pressure but has no nerve endings on its surface. Pain from the cervix usually feels like a bearing down sensation, sometimes with cramping. If you push the cervix gently with your finger you will find that it moves slightly. In fact the uterus changes position during sexual arousal and also at different stages of the menstrual cycle.

Doctors examine the cervix with the use of a speculum which is an instrument a little like a pair of tongs which is inserted closed into the vagina and then opened up to hold the walls of the vagina open so that the cervix can be inspected. There is a magnifying glass and often a light at the handle end. Many women find it helpful to examine themselves with a speculum. Cheap plastic speculums can be bought from any surgical supply shop. If you are interested in examining your cervix with a speculum, a detailed description of what to look for can be found in *The New Women's Health Handbook* edited by Nancy MacKeith.

The womb

During most of the last century it was believed by doctors that the womb was responsible for most of the ailments of the female sex, or at least those women who could afford to see a doctor. Generally these ailments came under the heading 'hysteria', a term which comes from the Greek word for uterus.

The symptoms of hysteria included agitation, convulsions, fainting fits, lassitude, violent screaming, crying or laughing as well as period pains and other such physical conditions. Most of these symptoms have since been taken into the steely arms of psychiatry but the legacy of this attitude to the womb lingers on in our feelings about menstruation, sex and birth. It is our hidden wombs which tie us to traditional womanhood. The more we understand about them, the better.

The uterus is a pear-shaped bag of muscle about the size of a clenched fist when in its non-pregnant state. It is domed at the top and narrows to a neck (the cervical canal and cervix) at the bottom. It is made of three strong layers of muscle woven together and is probably one of the most remarkable organs in the human body. Its elasticity is such that it can stretch from some 4 inches (9 cm) in length at conception to 20 inches (50 cm) when it cradles a full-grown foetus. It can then return to its original size within a matter of days after birth.

The muscles of the uterus are involuntary, that is, we cannot actually decide when we want to use them as we can

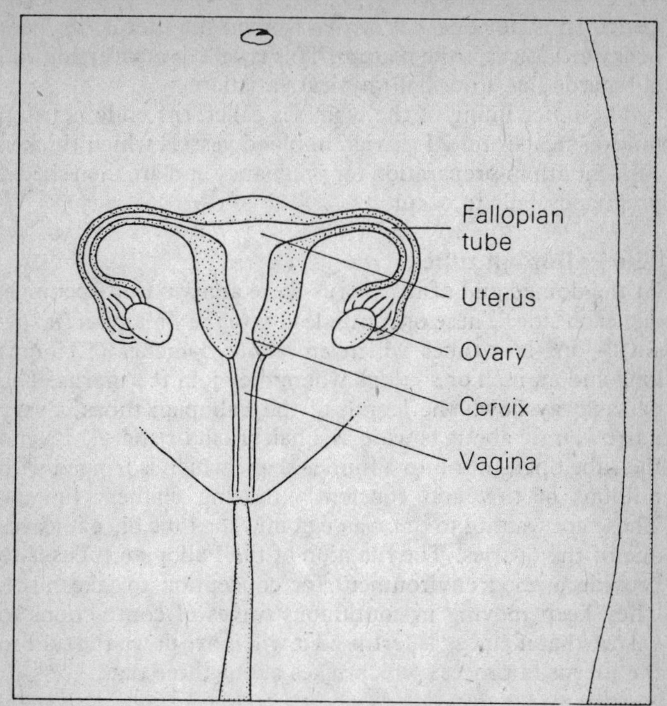

the muscles of the arms and legs. When they are triggered into action by hormones at the onset of labour they are, however, the strongest and most powerful muscles in the human body. Pain from the uterus is felt as cramps or backache or pain in the thighs. Period pains are typical of the pain felt by uterine contractions though why some women suffer from them and not others is still a mystery. In non-pregnant women there is a very narrow slit between the walls of the uterus which is called the uterine cavity. When you menstruate it is the lining of this cavity which is shed to produce blood.

The uterus is partially supported by strong, supple ligaments. It lies between the bladder and the rectum, normally at an angle of 90° to the vagina, resting on the bladder. When the bladder is full the uterus is pushed back and when the bladder is emptied the uterus drops forward again. In about one out of five women the uterus lies bent backward towards the rectum. This is called retroversion and is regarded as a normal physical variation.

The inner lining of the womb is called the endometrium (end-o-meat-rium). It is rich in blood vessels which thicken each month in preparation for pregnancy and are then shed if pregnancy fails to occur.

The Fallopian tubes

At the domed end of the uterus there are two tiny openings, one each side. These openings lead into the Fallopian (fal (as pal) – ope-ian) tubes which are about 5 inches (12.5 cm) long and an inch or so thick where they join the uterus. The passageway down the length of the Fallopian tubes is very narrow, only about as wide as a hairbrush bristle. At its end the tube opens out into a funnel-shape which is fringed with millions of tiny and constantly moving feathery fingers. These are waiting to draw an egg into the tube once it leaves one of the ovaries. The function of the Fallopian tubes is to provide a good environment for conception to take place. They keep moving in continuous waves of contractions to ensure that if an egg is fertilised it will move down the tube to the uterus, a process which takes about three days.

The ovaries

There are two ovaries which lie one on each side of the uterus and very close to the fringed fingers of the Fallopian tubes. They are both the warehouse for thousands of egg cells and also hormone factories which produce the female sex hormones oestrogen (east-row-jen) and progesterone (pro-jest-er-own). These are the hormones which control our reproductive cycle.

The ovaries are greyish white in colour and almond shaped. They are about 2 inches (4.5 cm) long and less than an inch (2.5 cm) thick. Their surface is covered by a tough white membrane. During each cycle one of the thousands of eggs in the ovary starts to ripen until it eventually breaks through this outer membrane and is caught by the fringed fingers of the Fallopian tube and drawn inside.

Chapter Two

Dealing with Doctors

In preparing my case
I parcelled up my worth
And threw it across
The communication gap
In the Doctor's surgery.

Some fool I was
That is what you do with God
At the desperate edge
Of the known,
Trying not to evaporate
In the hiatus.

Now I see you
Writing in your book
And you do not look
For parcels underfoot.

Anne Burge

It has been said that doctors are people we love to hate. Certainly as patients we indulge in much unofficial moaning even if we do little official complaining. The fact that we do moan is not a matter of national temperament or even human nature; it is more a reflection of the unsatisfactory nature of our relationship with doctors.

It is the inequality of the doctor-patient relationship which frustrates. Doctors possess information and skills which we need, yet they dispense these only as they see fit and we really have very little say in the matter. This is called 'clinical judgement'. It is very often a social judgement as well.

The individual personality of the doctor is obviously

important in this but the problem is more deep-rooted than that. It is inbuilt into the medical system that we are required to use. There are certain services which are vital to us and which are obtainable only through doctors. The most important of these are those facilities which effect our reproductive life and hence our freedom. Contraception, abortion, sterilisation and the maternity services are all controlled by doctors. And in these areas we are free to ignore them only at risk and inconvenience to ourselves. So we are compelled to play the system.

The system

The National Health Service was born shortly after the Second World War. The medical establishment attempted to abort the scheme but it was pushed through by a Labour government determined to ensure that medical services would be available free at the point of access to all who needed them. The NHS has since become a national institution second only to the monarchy in British affections.

The service is not free, of course, we pay for it through taxation. We put money into the system when we are healthy so that we can receive treatment during sickness. In fact the NHS is financed by potential patients, administered by the State bureaucracy and effectively shaped by its most powerful group of workers, the doctors.

The administration of the NHS is currently being re-organised yet again, the last effort in 1974 having proved cumbersome and unpopular. One of the tiers of the bureaucracy, the Regional Health Authorities, is to go and the Area Health Authorities are to be reorganised and called District Health Authorities. The boundaries of these are currently being discussed. So the administrative structure of the NHS will be as follows:

The man at the top is the Secretary of State for Social Services and his department is the Department of Health and Social Security (DHSS) Scottish Home and Health Department.

Next are the new *District Health Authorities* which are responsible for hospital services in the area and for making major decisions about the allocation of money or cutbacks in service. They are also responsible for complaints about hospital or community services.

Then there are the *Family Practitioner Committees*, one in each district, which are responsible for organising GP services, dealing with contracts and payment of GPs as well as complaints and disciplinary action.

The consumer voice is represented by the *Community Health Councils* whose function I will explain more fully later.

The doctor

The NHS employs nearly a million people of whom about 77,000 are doctors. By virtue of their position and prestige doctors have shaped the system to serve their best interests rather than the health needs of the population at large. Ninety per cent of illness occurs and is treated in the community, yet a disproportionate amount of money goes on technology for the ever-larger hospitals.

In recent years, however, the authority of the medical profession has come under attack both from the growing power of the unions representing other health service workers and from better-informed and critical patients. We no longer accept doctors who play god; we demand effective communication; we resent being patted on the head by our GP and we resent being treated as a serial number in a hospital bed. It is a confusing time for doctors and there is little in their training to help them.

Doctors are trained, over a period of six years, to be much the same as their teachers, the consultants in the great teaching hospitals, who specialise in narrow and often obscure areas of medicine and who hold enormous prestige within the profession itself. This is what is called 'real' medicine and the actual needs of the population for treatment in the areas of mental health and the chronic illnesses associated with old age are largely ignored. As one theory puts it, 'Doctors study medicine which they don't practise, and practise social science which they have not studied.'

In addition to this problem there is the fact that the majority of doctors do not come from the same class and are not the same sex as the majority of their patients. Most doctors come from the upper middle and middle classes. 20 per cent of medical students come from medical families. Only a little over 30 per cent of medical students are women and only 22 per cent of practising doctors. On the other hand, the majority of patients are female and working class.

The reason why there are more female patients is simply because there are more women in the population, especially among the older age groups. In addition, there are all the problems associated with a highly complicated reproductive system and the fact that women suffer from more social stress which leads them to seek help from their doctors.

Given the difference in upbringing, attitudes and lifestyle between the average male doctor and the average female patient, communication is obviously going to be difficult. Add to this the fact that medical students are selected for their academic ability not their human qualities and we are faced with a considerable, though not insurmountable, problem.

The general practitioner

> He's cold, unsympathetic, supercilious, condescending, patronising; he gives you the impression that you're a total bore, a hypochondriac and wasting his time.

> He listened to you. He somehow conveyed the feeling that help was there, he was there, which is what you need. He was an enormously humane man.

In the strictly medical area of diagnosis and treatment both these doctors were no doubt equally competent, but there is no question as to which surgery most of us would prefer to attend. Because, whilst the medical profession gives its highest honours for scientific and technical ability, most patients reserve their affection and respect for the humane and approachable doctor (provided, of course, that he isn't totally incompetent). And who can say we are wrong, for healing, after all, has been proved to be as much a matter of faith as of science. It is obviously very important to choose a GP you feel you can trust.

Choosing your doctor

Unfortunately, many people who move to a new area wait until they are ill before they register with a doctor and then they choose the one who practises down the road just because s/he practises down the road. Indeed, one GP told me: 'It's the experience of every doctor who moves premises a few hundred yards that plenty of patients won't come and see him because there's another doctor nearer.'

Be that as it may, the result is not usually very satisfactory. Research has shown that when people choose doctors in this haphazard way, one in five are dissatisfied with the one they choose. It is sensible to start looking for the right doctor as soon as you move, before you need medical attention.

If you live in a rural area or an inner city area there may not be very much choice, in which case you have to make the best of what's available. If there is a choice, however, you need to do your own consumer guide and it's not easy, because doctors in Britain are not permitted to advertise.

A list of all the doctors in your area should be available from the Post Office, Library, Citizens' Advice Bureau or Community Health Council or you can write to your local Family Practitioner Committee and ask them to send you a list. Unfortunately the list doesn't tell you very much about the doctors apart from name, address and telephone number, but it should indicate which ones are trained in obstetrics and will undertake maternity care and which ones are prepared to give contraceptive advice. You should also be able to see if there are any women doctors in the area if you want a woman doctor.

For further information you can look up the doctors in the medical directory in your library. This is a sort of *Who's Who* of the medical profession and will give you details of the doctors' careers and qualifications. But the best way of getting the low-down on doctors is to ask fellow consumers, neighbours, shopkeepers, in fact anyone you meet. Chemists are in a good position to know about doctors and are worth asking, as are health visitors if you have children. They may be reluctant to give advice but it is worth trying. It takes time to assess the different reports of different doctors and to judge for yourself which one you feel would most suit you but it's important to do it. Believe me, I speak from bitter experience!

Once you have selected a doctor you think sounds right you should ask the receptionist if you can talk to the doctor *before* registering. It won't always work, of course, some doctors object to the idea of being interviewed by potential patients and others are just too busy:

> I don't particularly welcome it, I'm too busy. I've got a number of friends who do say, 'If people want to come and register with me, I will interview them and we will discuss what they want out of me.' I think that's a very nice idea and I would like to have time to do it but I simply don't. I get enough people wanting to register to make my list up and I spend a lot of time turning people away because we're full.

The doctor who told me this was concerned about his relationship with his patients but he worked in an inner city area with a highly mobile population. If the doctor won't see you first you can always try for a temporary registration as you would if you were on holiday. A temporary registration lasts for a period of up to three months. Again, the receptionist may give you short shrift, in which case you have to decide whether to register anyway on the information you've been given or whether to try elsewhere.

If the doctor agrees to an interview, it's a good idea to write down on a piece of paper the questions you want to ask. This is a good general principle for all consultations with doctors because it's very easy to forget in the fluster of the moment what you really want to know. The kind of things you will probably be looking for from your doctor are:

1. His or her attitude to home visits. Some doctors are unwilling to visit except in emergencies.
2. His or her attitude to contraceptives, abortion or home confinement (if this is relevant to you).
3. Is there an appointment system and if so, how flexible is it?
4. Does s/he use a deputising service for evening calls?

5. Will it be possible to see the same doctor if there is a group practice?
6. Is s/he interested in gynaecology? GPs tend to have specialist interests and it's useful to find out what they are.

These are only a few of the things you may want to know. Ask what seems relevant to you. If you have any strong views or information about your history tell the doctor at this interview so that s/he will also have some knowledge about *you*.

Doctors see many more different people in the course of a working day than patients see doctors, so they are much better at handling these interviews. It is important for you to watch the way in which s/he handles your questions. If s/he has a sense of humour it's a plus; if s/he seems irritable and avoids looking at you, beware.

Once you have decided which doctor you wish to register with and s/he has accepted you, then you simply sign part A on your medical card and give it to the receptionist. The doctor will then sign the card, send it to the Family Practitioner Committee and they will send you a new one.

Talking to doctors

It can be difficult to talk to your doctor either because the problem is embarrassing or because you don't know quite how to explain what is wrong. It is always a good idea to prepare yourself beforehand by writing down a list of all your symptoms and a list of all the questions you want answered about them. Explain clearly to the doctor what you think is wrong with you, how you feel about it and what you hope can be done about it. If the doctor seems evasive, don't be put off, keep asking calmly and politely until you receive the answers that satisfy you.

If the doctor eventually writes you a prescription (which these days seems to be the inevitable conclusion to most medical consultations) then it is worth asking what the drug will do, whether it will have any side effects, whether it is safe to take with any other drugs (including alcohol), how quickly it will take effect and whether there are any alternative treatments.

If the treatment you receive is complicated or if you need a lengthy explanation of your problem, then it is worth writing notes so that you don't forget what has been said. Research shows that people remember the first and last points their doctors make and tend to forget everything in between. This may explain why 30 per cent of people fail to follow their doctors' instructions about prescribed drugs. Drugs are dangerous substances, it is always important to take them correctly.

If you are unhappy about the treatment your doctor recommends, say so, and explain your reasons. If you feel his or her diagnosis might be wrong, ask if there might be an alternative diagnosis. Your doctor is your expert adviser but s/he is not infallible and s/he does not know *your* body as well as you do. It is *your* body, *your* life, *your* health that is under discussion; you should take the ultimate responsibility for it. A good doctor will always be prepared to answer questions as well as s/he can, but doctors aren't mind readers and if you don't ask questions they are likely to assume that you aren't interested.

Of course many doctors take the professional attitude, 'I know best, leave it all to me and just do as you're told.' And this isn't easy to combat. But it can be done with practice. If you fail the first time, don't give up. You need to let your doctor know that you are *really* interested in sharing responsibility for your health. Challenging his or her authority seems frightening but it's necessary and each small success leads to greater confidence. It can often lead to a good relationship. If it leads to a bad one you must change your doctor.

Changing your doctor

The contract between doctor and patient can be ended by either party. If your doctor decides to remove you from his list he need give no reason though the implication will be that you are a difficult patient and this may make it hard for you to find another doctor. It is not a satisfactory situation, as one Community Health Councillor told me:

> The great problem with GPs is that once it's known that you've made any sort of bleat of complaint, you're off their books. So it really militates against anybody complaining. In other words I suggest that people put up with an awful lot.

It's a game where doctors hold most of the cards and they know it. This is why it is so important to find the right doctor in the first place. It *is* possible to change doctors within your area, however, and if you feel that you no longer have any faith in your GP it is important that you find another.

If you are moving house within the area, even if it is to another house in the same street, then you can register with a new doctor without any problems. If you're not, however, then you have to accept that doctors are understandably reluctant to be seen taking patients from each other:

> It's a bit hard for me, you see . . . I don't mind usually, but if someone comes in and says, 'Look, I want to change because I can't stand Dr X,' and I accept them, then Dr X is likely to feel a bit cross about it.

Within Health Centres the situation can be even more difficult:

> Within the Health Centre we don't accept patients from doctors who are within our own rota. If a patient leaves Dr X to come onto our books, for instance, and then encounters Dr X on a Sunday, it would be *very* embarrassing for both sides.

So it is wise to try and find out as much as possible about the way the doctor you hope to move to works before you approach him or her. It is also important to make sure that s/he is still accepting new patients. Then write to the Family Practitioner Committee (the address is on your medical card) and tell them that you no longer wish to be a patient of Dr X. You can then go to your new doctor and tell him or her that you have no GP and s/he need not fear being seen to steal patients.

It's a bore but it's better than putting up with a bad relationship. Most reasonable doctors recognise that there are valid reasons for patients to want to change:

> There are practices near me from whom I get a continuous, significant number of people who want to change. And having listened to what these people say and even allowing for the degree of bias that always creeps into these stories, I'm confident that I'm getting a fairly accurate picture of what goes on, which is confirmed by the notes when they arrive two months later.

> I can see that the girl who's got an older GP who knows her parents would have problems. They don't want to go and talk to their parents' friend about their pills or their babies or their sex life. They just want to go somewhere else.

> We would accept patients who feel they want to change to a woman doctor.

> We tend to know our colleagues. We tend to know that some of our colleagues are dismissive about coughs and colds and suchlike. Some doctors don't go out to visit and we know that too. So there are circumstances when we would accept patients.

These are just a few comments from doctors I asked about this, but they show a refreshing degree of awareness and realism.

Once you have been accepted by your new doctor, you have two options.

You can ask your old doctor to sign part B on your medical card giving his or her consent to change. You then complete the details on the card and take it to your new doctor who will sign part A and send it to the Family Practitioner Committee.

If you'd prefer not to see your old doctor again, and it can be embarrassing, then you send your card to the Family Practitioner Committee informing them that you wish to change doctors. You do not need to explain why you want to change. If you have been accepted by your new doctor give his or her name. You will not be allowed to transfer until at least fourteen days after the Committee receives your letter. (This delay is supposed to prevent patients from changing doctors too often.) The FPC will return your card with a slip which has to be completed and taken to your new doctor who will do the rest.

If for some reason you are unable to find a doctor who will accept you, then you should write to the FPC telling them which doctors have refused you. The FPC have a duty to provide a doctor for anybody who wants one who is living in the area. So they will allocate a doctor. It may not be the doctor you wanted or one that's reasonably close to where you live but at least you will have medical cover.

Specialists

Specialist doctors work exclusively in hospitals or private practice or both. They are doctors who have specialised in treating a certain area or certain organs of the human body. The specialists you are most likely to see if you suffer from problems below the belt are:

Gynaecologist (g-eye-knee-col-o-jist) A doctor who is trained to deal with our sexual and reproductive organs. Since most gynaecologists are male they don't always see things the way we do.

Obstetrician (ob-stet-rishian) A doctor usually trained as a gynaecologist but specialising in antenatal care and the delivery of babies.

Urologist (yur-ol-ogist) A doctor who specialises in the disorders and diseases of the urinary system (kidneys, ureters, bladder and urethra).

Venereologist (ven-ear-eol-ogist) A doctor who specialises in the diagnosis and treatment of sexually transmitted diseases.

The main snag about specialists is that you can normally see them only if your GP decides that you need to. As one woman told me:

What really annoys me is that you have to fight to get a letter to go and see a specialist. My doctor just said, 'They can't do anything or give you anything that I can't give you,' and he *refused*. So I had to go round him.

It is not an ideal situation to have to bypass your GP but it can be done. If you feel that your GP is not giving your complaint the attention it deserves, then you can go and be checked at one of the following clinics. Some women do this all the time, though it is better to change your GP if things get this bad:

> I had one friend who just had to give up going to the doctor altogether and has to use local authority clinics until she can get on another list because her doctor is a complete imbecile and can't diagnose anything, can't treat anything and refuses to refer her to anyone.

Well-Women clinics

These provide a kind of gynaecological MOT test. You will have your blood pressure and urine checked, breast and vaginal examinations and a cervical smear test done. It is part of their policy to try and and use female staff so if you find it difficult to discuss personal or sexual matters with a male GP you may find it easier to approach one of the female doctors at this clinic. Many of us also find the impersonal atmosphere of a clinic less stressful when it comes to discussing parts of our body we find embarrassing. After all, you won't have to face the doctor again next week when the toddler gets tonsillitis.

If you are worried about a persistent pain or discharge and your GP will not examine you or refer you to a gynaecologist, then it is worth going to a Well-Women clinic to be checked. If the clinic finds something wrong they should inform your GP who will then be under much greater pressure to refer.

Special Clinics

If you have any reason to suspect that you might have a sexually transmitted disease then it is wise to go to a special clinic for a check-up. You will receive a more thorough check-up. You will receive a more thorough check-up at one of these

properly. I now eat a wholefood diet and I'm finding that I feel a lot healthier, I've got more energy.

Most alternative forms of medicine are not available on the National Health. Homeopathy is, however. Homeopathic doctors are trained to treat the whole patient rather than the symptoms. The natural medicines are tailored individually but the basic principle is to treat a patient's symptoms with a medicine which would create those symptoms in a healthy person. In most cases it seems to be beneficial.

Other alternatives to conventional medicine exist in the form of self-help and women's health groups. These are enormously helpful in providing both support and basic information. Once people start taking responsibility for their own health and learning more about how their bodies work they are able to make more effective demands on the health system.

Useful addresses

Homeopathy: contact the *British Homeopathic Association* 27a Devonshire Street, London W1 for a list of practitioners.
Naturopathy: contact the *British Naturopathic and Osteopathic Association* 6 Netherhall Gardens, London NW3 for a list of practitioners.
Acupuncture: contact the *Acupuncture Association and Register* for a list of practitioners.
Women's health groups: contact WIRES 32a Shakespeare St, Nottingham for information about any local groups.

Chapter Three

The Curse

We bleed regularly. Regularly each month for the best part of forty years we bleed. It is called menstruation, a word which comes from the Latin mens-mensis meaning month. Month means 'the moon's period'. Magical. Not that most of us see much that is magical about our periods but the cycle of death and renewal is there whether we like it or not.

Most cultures have treated menstruation as a magical time and a time especially dangerous to men. For this reason numerous taboos and superstitions have been built around the time of bleeding. In many societies women were forced to withdraw and hide at this time in special huts, for it was believed that menstruating women would wither young plants, poison meat, make milk sour and even bring death. And if in modern western society we are no longer expected to hide ourselves, we are expected to hide our bleeding. All advertisements for sanitary pads and tampons emphasise their secrecy. Women who talk quite freely about sex become embarrassed when asked about their periods. The bleeding is shameful, unclean, the nightmare is to be discovered, especially by men:

> She dreamt she was in the room where orals were held, a wood-paneled room with small paned windows and a broad shining table ... She had just stepped inside the door when she spied the pile in the corner. Instantly she knew what it was, but she was incredulous, she was so ashamed, she moved nearer to check it out. It was what she thought. She was horrified. Those stained sanitary napkins, those bloody underpants were hers, and she knew the men would know it too.

This, written by Marilyn French in *The Women's Room*, is probably the kind of nightmare most of us have had at one time or another. So the mythology hangs on, and the idea that it is dangerous to go swimming or walk barefoot on cold floors or even wash your hair whilst menstruating still persist though there is no truth in them.

It all comes down to education in the end. The way that we feel about our bodies springs from the way we come to learn about their functioning, the feelings we pick up from our mothers and older women, whispers in the school playground. One woman I talked to was told by a friend when she saw a bloody sanitary pad in the school toilets that if she ever needed one of those she wouldn't be able to have babies. Another woman, in her early twenties, told me:

> I started my periods when I was nine which was a bit awkward because nobody bothered to tell me anything about these things and I was quite convinced I was bleeding to death. I didn't have a clue what it was about.

And so it goes, variations on the same theme, endlessly repeated. Small wonder that menstruation is called the curse and puberty is such a trauma. In an ideal world young girls would be told about their bodies in a simple, factual way and in a loving, informal atmosphere.

Puberty (the menarche)

Puberty is the time when girls become women. The reproductive system matures under the influence of increased hormonal activity and the familiar female shape develops from the childish body. No one really understands how the brain decides the time is right to start the circulation of hormones in the body which produces these changes. There is, however, some relationship between the start of puberty and body weight, for puberty starts in most of us when we weigh about 6½–7 stone. This might explain why the age at which puberty starts varies so much.

Puberty has been starting earlier and earlier over the past hundred years. In 1850 the average age for the start of the first period (the menarche) was 17.5 years, in 1976 the average was found to be 12.8 years with a range between 10.4 and 15.2 years. This change is accounted for by the fact that we eat rather better than we used to.

The hormonal changes which trigger puberty are fairly complicated but worth knowing. It all starts with a part of the brain called the *hypothalmus*. This part of the brain not only sends messages to the hormone system, it is also capable of responding to messages from the nervous system which probably explains the connection between emotional stress and irregular periods.

The hypothalmus makes and sends out special hormones direct to a gland in the middle of the brain called the *pituitary* gland. This gland is responsible for sending out a number of hormones but the two which affect our reproductive cycle are known by the initials FSH (follicle stimulating hormone) and LH (luteinising hormone.) FSH is first directed into the system to stir the ovaries into action and as the immature ovaries begin to grow they also begin to secrete the sex hormone oestrogen. As the body's level of oestrogen rises, so the sex changes begin and young women enter puberty.

The development of the breast nipple is the first obvious sign of puberty, followed later by growth of the breast itself. At the same time as this is happening the sexual organs grow and the lining of the uterus starts to thicken. Over the hips and thighs appear the fat deposits we are all so familiar with. All this is accompanied by a considerable growth spurt. Next the body hair begins to grow and acne may start to develop. By the time the young woman has pubic hair and fairly well developed breasts she may expect to experience her first menstrual period.

In many cultures the menarche is greeted with initiation ceremonies, not all of which are pleasant. In western society it is usually hidden, like all other aspects of menstruation. The subject is less hidden than it used to be but on the whole young women are still left to handle the transition on their own.

The first period usually lasts between three and eight days and there may be a gap of two or three months before the next one. Periods are usually so irregular to begin with because ovulation has not yet started. At some stage after the first period the pituitary gland begins to secrete LH which stimulates ovulation, or the release of the egg from the ovary and into the Fallopian tube. It is impossible to say at exactly what point this happens, it may be anything up to two years after the first period but it is unwise to rely on it as a contraceptive. Once ovulation starts menstruation normally settles down to a regular and more frequent cycle.

The menstrual cycle

Our reproductive cycle works under the influence of hormones. First FSH is released which stimulates the ovary to produced follicles or tiny protective bags containing unripe eggs. These follicles appear on the surface of the ovary rather like little bubbles, though normally only one of them will burst to produce a ripe egg. Whilst this is happening the ovaries are producing increased quantities of oestrogen which stirs the uterus into preparing a thick lining ready to nourish any fertilised egg. Somewhere in the middle of the cycle the levels of oestrogen reach a point where the pituitary gland is triggered into sending out the second hormone, LH, which makes the follicle burst and release its ripe egg. Some women can actually feel this happen. Once the egg has been released it is caught by the fingers of the Fallopian tube and begins its journey down the tube where it may or may not be fertilised.

Once ovulation has occurred, the empty follicle collapses and the follicle cells rearrange themselves under the influence of LH. They continue to produce oestrogen but now begin to produce the other female sex hormone, progesterone, as well. The name progesterone means pro-gestation or pro-pregnancy and it works on the lining of the uterus ensuring it will be prepared to nourish a fertilised egg.

If conception does not take place, then the body's levels of oestrogen and progesterone drop, the stimulus to the uterus ceases and so the lining separates from the wall of the uterus and we bleed. Then the process starts all over again.

You will notice that this hormone cycle also affects the mucus discharged from the cervix into the vagina. During the early days of the cycle there is very little mucus but as the oestrogen level rises, so the amount of mucus increases. At the time of ovulation there is a great deal and it is wet, stringy and elastic. After ovulation, under the influence of progesterone, it becomes thick and sticky and there is less of it. Then following the bleeding there is very little of it again.

Normal menstruation

Women vary so much that normal menstruation means about as much as normal height or normal weight. The average length of the menstrual cycle is usually given as 28 days, but that is very much an average. You measure your menstrual cycle from the first day of bleeding to the last day before the bleeding of the next cycle. This may be anything from twenty-one to thirty-five days.

The bleeding itself may last for as little as three days or go on for as long as eight days, all of which is quite normal. The important thing is to establish what is normal for *you* and worry only if your particular cycle starts changing. The same holds true for the amount of blood lost. If we say we have had a 'heavy' period, we can only mean that it has been heavy for us, since we have no way of knowing how much blood other women lose. If we do start losing an inconveniently heavy amount, then it is always worth checking to ensure nothing is wrong.

Period pains (dysmenorrhoea)

About half of all women suffer from some pain at the start of a period. For most it is tolerable and can be coped with by taking aspirin or paracetemol. But for some women it is absolute agony, with severe pains much like labour pains, together with nausea, dizziness and fainting. As one woman told me:

> I used to start my period in the middle of the night, always. I used to wake up in absolute agony and the pain was so intense that I couldn't lie still and I would literally writhe around in bed. The pain lasted for the first day. I used to end up in bed with hot water bottles and tablets, if I could keep them down, because I used to just vomit.

Another woman remembered much the same thing:

> When a period started, I had very bad period cramps. I remember sort of lying on the floor screaming and things like that. I don't remember at the beginning being given anything to relieve the pain, but later I found there were pills I could take that would make it quite bearable.

Period pains like these are called primary or spasmodic *dysmenorrhoea* (dis-men-ore-ear), they come regularly every cycle and are usually worst for the first 24 to 36 hours of the period. They begin soon after periods have become established in the teens and if there is no pregnancy they often tail off gradually after the age of 25. If there has been a pregnancy period pains may cease completely. Doctors are prone to tell young teenagers not to worry, and that it'll clear up when they've had a baby, which is cold comfort and not always true.

No one really knows why we suffer from period pains. It is possible that we simply aren't physically adapted to having periods so often. After all, most women in history have been tied to a cycle of constant pregnancies and breastfeeding from a very young age. It is only in recent history that we have had the means to free ourselves from our biology.

It used to be believed that period pains were self-induced, neurotic, a sign of inherent weakness, an excuse for avoiding work and a means of getting attention. There are still some doctors, usually the older ones, who believe this. If you have such a doctor it would seem a good idea to find a new one or go to a Well-Woman or family planning clinic for attention. There is no need to suffer in silence.

Current theories tend to emphasise hormonal imbalance of one kind or another as the cause. Only time will tell whether these theories are accurate but at least we know that one way to completely clear period pains is to go on the contraceptive pill. Whether this is an acceptable treatment for a young woman, of course, is a different matter, since the pill has dangers of its own. It is always a question of balancing risks.

Sometimes period pains can be caused by a medical

problem such as pelvic infection, fibroids or endometriosis. Cramps caused by such conditions are called secondary dysmenhorrhea but they feel much the same. So it is important to be examined if you go to the doctor because of period pains and a good doctor should do this. One I talked to explained:

> I don't usually prescribe the pill for dysmenhorrea without a specialist opinion, unless I know what's going on. There could be a medical reason and I think the pill's a bit of a blanket sometimes. So I think unless she's been examined one ought not just to stick her on the pill.

Another and more drastic method of dealing with menstrual pains is the surgical operation known as D&C (Dilation and Curettage) which involves the widening of the cervix and scraping of the lining of the uterus. This can be effective for a short time but some women find the pains return, as this woman did:

> I had a D&C when I was 21 but the pains came back and then when I was 24 it was so bad I found it difficult to work so I had another D&C. Again, that worked for a few months and then it started to revert back to normal.

Alternative remedies

Diet Making sure that you eat the right food can often help. Avoid eating spicy foods and too much salt during the week before your period and try to stick to a high protein and low sugar diet. Vegetable protein is supposed to be especially helpful so try and eat plenty of fresh vegetables.

Exercises There are exercises which can help to ease period pains, especially relaxation exercises.

Find a really comfortable position to lie in with pillows under your head and shoulders and a pillow under your knees. Clench both fists very hard and take a deep breath through your nose. Breathe out slowly through your mouth until your lungs are completely empty and at the same time let your hands fall loosely. Try this two or three times at first. Your hands should feel very heavy. Relaxation is something which improves with practise, so don't give up if it doesn't happen at once.

Next try the same exercise, tensing and relaxing your feet and ankles and then your shoulders and face. Remember to keep the breathing pattern the same. Concentrate on keeping your mouth loose, there is a curious connection betwen the muscles of the mouth and those of the vagina. When your whole body is completely relaxed you will find that it feels heavy and warm and you may well fall off to sleep.

Another good exercise is to lie on your back and lean your feet up against a wall so that they are higher than your head. Again, make sure that you are comfortable and keep in this position for five or ten minutes. It is a general rule that women who take regular exercise like walking, running or swimming, tend to suffer less from period pains, so it is a good idea to try and keep as fit as possible all the time.

Sex Many women find that having orgasms is a good way to relieve period pains since it increases the blood flow to the pelvic area and seems to make the uterus relax. If you don't feel like having sex with a partner, an orgasm achieved through masturbation is just as effective.

In addition to these self-help treatments, some women find meditation, yoga, herbal remedies or acupuncture have been useful.

Having No Periods (amenorrhoea)

The commonest reason for periods stopping is pregnancy, so although not having periods is not actually dangerous, it can be worrying unless you are quite positive that you can't be pregnant.

There are a number of quite straightforward reasons why we may miss a period. It usually happens because something has upset the normal hormone cycle. Women who stop taking the pill often find that they go without periods for a few months. If this happens it doesn't mean you can't get pregnant, so do take precautions if you don't want a baby.

Stress can also effect menstruation. If you suffer from a sudden shock like an accident or a bereavement your periods may stop for many weeks. If you are working in a stressful job or upset by a crumbling relationship it may also effect your cycle. If this happens it is worth thinking carefully about your situation to see if you can change anything to make life more relaxed. Your periods should return once the shock or stress has passed.

Diet is another factor responsible for stopping menstruation. If your weight drops below about 7 stone (48 kilos) then your periods may cease. Women who were prisoners in the Japanese camps during the last war with a combination of stress and poor diet stopped menstruating for years. Today women who suffer from anorexia nervosa often have no periods, but it can equally well happen if you diet too enthusiastically:

> I was about 17 and I had been on a strict diet. I wasn't anorexic, I had to fight to keep on this diet because I wanted to be terribly thin, and I stopped getting my periods. That when on for about four or five months until finally I went to the doctor and she said, 'Have you been on a diet?'

Diseases such as tuberculosis, anaemia, rheumatic fever, acute depression and certain thyroid problems can also halt menstruation. So too can some anti-depressant drugs and certain drugs given for high blood pressure. If you suffer from delayed menstruation and are concerned about any drugs you are taking, ask your doctor about it.

Usually periods return on their own but if you have not been menstruating for five months or so then it is sensible to visit your doctor. Never take any drug treatment designed to bring your periods back until you have had a pregnancy test since these drugs can harm the foetus.

Bleeding too much (menorrhagia)

Sometimes periods go on for longer than usual or are heavier than usual or come more often. If the change is sudden and upsetting it is worth checking with your doctor as it *may* mean there is something wrong. The most common reasons for heavy or prolonged periods are polyps or fibroids (see Chapter 10). Many women also experience heavy bleeding when they have an IUD or coil.

If you have a regular cycle and you start having irregular bleeding or 'spotting' between periods then it should be checked by a doctor. It might indicate an early stage of cervical cancer (see Chapter 9) which can be treated if caught at this stage.

If you are approaching the menopause you may find that your cycle starts going haywire. Generally the cycle will be shorter but whilst some women bleed more and for longer others find they bleed less for a shorter time. If you are worried or find your periods inconveniently heavy don't suffer in silence.

The Menopause

We live in a youth-oriented culture where middle age is viewed as a decline and the menopause the end. It is all nonsense, of course, since the menopause marks only the end of fertility and is often the beginning of a new phase of sexuality. This is a time when many women feel released from all the problems of their menstrual cycle and fears about unwanted pregnancy and the dangers of contraception. If we try and think positively about ourselves and our bodies at this time a new and more liberated sexuality can develop. But it isn't always easy for the middle years are a time of social and emotional as well as physical change; a time for re-assessing our self image as the children leave home and our body image as our fertile years come to an end.

As we approach the menopause, our ovaries stop producing their egg each month and there is a decline in the amount of oestrogen and progesterone they produce. This process normally occurs between the ages of 48 and 52 but it can start as early as 35 or as late as 56.

There are certain physical problems associated with the menopause though these again vary between women. The two most common symptoms are 'hot flushes' and loss of elasticity and moisture in the vagina. A hot flush is a sudden sensation of heat in the top part of the body. It lasts several seconds, may produce sweating and usually occurs at night. Their cause is not really understood but it is probably the body's attempt to adjust to reduced hormone levels as the menstrual cycle winds down. The drop in hormone levels also means that the vagina secretes less fluid and becomes drier and less stretchy. If this makes intercourse difficult and uncomfortable a lubricant such as KY jelly usually works very well.

A few women experience other problems such as palpitations and dizziness and there may be a general feeling of tiredness which is probably as much a result of nights disturbed by hot flushes as anything else.

Menopausal symptoms can be treated medically by hormone replacement therapy (HRT) which usually involves taking oestrogen (or more rarely progesterone) in the form of pills, injections or implants. This treatment can be very effective and was hailed as *the* answer to menopausal miseries a few years ago. It has since been discovered that the treatment has been associated with an increase in endometrial cancer since when it has been viewed with more caution.

Hormones have a considerable effect on the body, as was discovered with the Pill, and it is not entirely understood how they work. There is considerable controversy over the use of HRT and it is a difficult area to make sense of. Certainly most cases of vaginal dryness and hot flushes are eased by oestrogen therapy. On the other hand, it is known that taking oestrogen increases the risk of blood clots, heart disease and high blood pressure. Some women taking oestrogen experience stomach upsets, water retention, weight gain, headaches, vaginal discharge and changes in skin pigmentation but the kind of side effects varies with the kind of oestrogen taken.

If your life is made a misery by your menopausal symptoms, then it is probably wise to have a long discussion with your doctor to find out exactly what the benefits and risks might be in *your* case. Since the scientific evidence from research studies is still not conclusive, this is one of those areas, like whooping cough immunisation, where you have to try and assess the risks for yourself.

Old fashioned doctors can still be very unsympathetic about menopausal symptoms. It is, again, an area where men have no actual experience and therefore easily assume you're making a fuss about nothing. Don't allow yourself to be dismissed as neurotic, treatments are available and should be discussed. It is your body and you have a right to be involved in decisions made about it.

Alternative treatments are available. Some women find that natural homeopathic remedies or herbal cures are helpful (see bibliography at the end of the book). Others use relaxation exercises or yoga. It is known that hot flushes can be provoked by hot tea and coffee and by eating spicy foods, so these should be avoided. Certainly a good diet and sensible exercise throughout your thirties will help your body to adjust more easily to the hormonal changes.

Tampon Shock Syndrome

News has recently come from America that no less than 17 deaths have been associated with the use of tampons.

The symptoms are vomiting and diarrhoea with a very high temperature, intense muscle pain, a bright red rash and a rapid drop in blood pressure.

The cause seems to be the new 'super-absorbent' tampons which are made from synthetic fibres. It is thought that these may become a breeding ground for bacteria in the vagina though no one is entirely sure how this might happen. There is also concern about the chemicals used to deodorise and hold together the new fibres. It is thought that the plastic applicators of some new brands are more likely to scratch the vagina and introduce these chemicals into the bloodstream. It is unwise and unnecessary ever to use deodorised tampons and it is better to avoid new makes with synthetic fibres. Sanitary pads still seem to be safe.

An alternative to the expense and risk of tampons (and all sanitary towels carry VAT) is to use a natural sponge instead. You can buy small natural sponges, and they *must* be natural, not synthetic, from the baby counter at most large chemists.

Choose one which has small holes. Wet the sponge well with warm water, squeeze it dry, then insert it in the vagina. It is as absorbant as any tampon. Each time you go to the toilet, remove the sponge and rinse it through in cool, running water (hot water will stain it.)

Sponges are very comfortable and soft to wear and are much cheaper than buying packs of sanitary pads. There are also no problems of disposal. If you buy two sponges you will always have a spare in case of emergencies. To ensure that they are always clean, keep them stored in a very weak solution of Savlon (about one teaspoon to a pint) in a jar. When you use them, ensure that you rinse them very, very thoroughly in cool water to remove as much of the disinfectant as possible. Disinfectant should not be introduced into the vagina. Natural sponge should never be boiled or it will disintegrate.

Menstruation still retains many mysteries. Women who live closely together for any length of time will synchronise their menstrual cycles so that they bleed together. This has been noticed not only in women's prisons but in the ordinary home where mother and daughter share the same cycle. It is thought that there may be some connection with that most neglected of senses, scent. Nor do we really understand why our feelings are affected so much by the menstrual cycle, a subject which is discussed in the next chapter.

Chapter Four

Premenstrual Tension

There's a joke that runs: 'After all the publicity I thought I'd better develop premenstrual tension.' It's not a very funny joke. It's not a very funny condition:

> It really is so bad that it affects my life. I *cannot* stand noise and things like that. I'm just so bad tempered. And I start breaking things. It'll all happen in say the space of three or four days. I'll break several things and then I'll go on for weeks and not break anything.
>
> My husband says it's totally predictable. I start snapping. I tense up. I don't think I'd call it depression but it is tension. I start sleeping badly. I tend to wake up very early in the morning and get very uptight because I'm tired and it builds up. I'm always convinced I'm going to have lung cancer and everything else in that week and I always want to do drastic things like moving house. I never feel I can cope with anything.

Neither of these women suffer from really severe premenstrual tension yet both are sufficiently affected to find it dreary and a drag. Others find it quite incapacitating and it can be dangerous if a woman becomes too accident prone. The publicity which has surrounded the subject has been necessary because, like most women's problems, this one has been neglected and dismissed:

> It's only because premenstrual tension has suddenly become a topical subject that you start to think about it and you work out your dates and realise that it's always that time of month that you're incredibly bad tempered and

then you understand why and that there's something you can do about it.

Premenstrual tension (usually known as PMT) is actually only one of the symptoms of what is more correctly called the *premenstrual syndrome.* A syndrome is a characteristic group of symptoms and the special character of this particular group of symptoms is that they occur each month in the days or weeks before menstruation.

Symptoms

The important thing to remember about these symptoms is that they occur only before menstruation and not at other times of the month. So it is important to keep a menstrual chart so that you can check that your symptoms are definitely connected with your periods. Physical symptoms include:

Headaches: these may vary from tension headaches which feel like a cap of steel pressing on your head to full migraine headaches which may include nausea and vomiting. Women who suffer from premenstrual headaches often find they become worse if they are on the pill. On the other hand they are likely to stop during the last part of pregnancy and after the menopause.

Water retention: this includes swelling of the abdomen, ankles and fingers; tender and swollen breasts and a pattern of weight gain as the period approaches, all of which is accompanied by a general feeling of heaviness and bloatedness. Sufferers find that the symptoms are usually worse in the morning. It is important to realise that your weight gain is due to water being retained in your body *not* to fat. Try to limit your fluids to four cups a day and cut down on salt in your diet. This will help far more than cutting down on food which can, in fact, make things worse.

Muscle pains: these include backache, cramps and general aches and pains in the joints.

Skin disorders: including acne, pimples, styes, boils and herpes.

Some women suffer from premenstrual attacks of asthma or epilepsy. Some suffer from dizziness, fainting or find they are especially prone to cystitis during the premenstrual period. It is thought that many of these physical symptoms are related to the fact that too much water is retained in the body instead of being removed by the kidneys. Mental symptoms include:

Poor concentration: this may involve such things as insomnia, forgetfulness, finding you are easily distracted or finding it difficult to make sensible decisions.

Irritability and depression: very often weepiness and tetchiness go together. Everything seems wrong and you lash out at the least thing. Sometimes there may be attacks of anxiety.

Tiredness: many women feel tired, apathetic and listless before their period. If this happens it can effect your efficiency at work and your ability to get through the most routine housework. Schoolgirls and students may find their mental agility effected by this tiredness which can be a real worry at exam time.

When it happens

Women suffer from different combinations of these symptoms with varying degrees of severity. Each woman also has her own cyclic pattern: 'It starts about five days before I menstruate and it carries on until I start menstruating heavily. It's about a week,' one woman told me, and her pattern is probably the most common. Some women find it lasts rather longer, however, and others suffer for only a day or so.

It is important to establish exactly what your pattern is to ensure that your problems are indeed due to the premenstrual syndrome and not to something else. Premenstrual symptoms occur only in the days before your period and the rest of the month you should be completely symptom free. In order to see clearly whether this is the case, the simplest thing to do is to keep a menstrual chart.

Two examples of menstrual charts are shown here. The first shows the cycle of a premenstrual tension sufferer and the second shows a chart with symptoms unrelated to menstruation.

	June	July	Aug	Sept
1			T+P	
2			P	
3		T	P	
4		T	P	
5		T+A	P	
6		T+A		
7		T+P		
8		P		
9		P		
10	T+A	P		
11	T+A	P		T+A
12	T+A			T
13	T			T
14	T+P			T
15	P			T+P
16	P			P
17	P			P
18	P			P
19				P
20				
21				
22			T+A	
23			T+A	
24			T	
25			T	
26			T+P	
27		T	P	
28		T	P	
29		T	P	
30		T	P	
31		T		

PMT sufferer

P = period　　T = tension
H = headache　　A = accident

	June	July	Aug	Sept
1				P
2				P
3				P
4	H			P
5			P	
6		H	P	
7			P	
8			P	
9	H	P	P	
10		P		
11		P		H+T
12		P		T
13		P		
14	P			
15	P			
16	P			
17	P			
18	P			
19			H	
20			H	
21				
22				
23				
24				P
25				P
26				P
27				P
28				P
29				
30				
31			P	

unrelated symptoms

P = period T = tension
H = headache A = accident

Most women choose to use the first letter of the symptom on their chart, H for headache, B for backache, A for accidents and so on, but any letters or symbols can be used provided you remember what they mean. You will find that it is much easier to organise your life if you know when to expect premenstrual symptoms and how to work round them.

The premenstrual syndrome does not necessarily begin when you start your periods, indeed many women only notice it after they have had children:

> I had no problems whatsoever until I had children; none that I was aware of. I think it started after I had my first baby though I don't think I realised what it was, initially, so I probably didn't look at it in relation to the monthly cycle. I became more aware of it with the second child. I saw a pattern.

Whether premenstrual symptoms do in fact get worse after having baby or whether we simply notice them more because we are under more stress is a difficult question:

> It seems to have got worse after each baby. I say got worse, I'm more aware of it now. Things happen as you get older; you become aware of things like that which you've not talked about before to other people.

Certainly it has been found that if a woman suffers from postnatal depression there is a 90 per cent chance of the premenstrual syndrome subsequently developing. Whether this is due to hormonal imbalance or psychological stress or an interaction between the two is a matter of debate.

The Social Effect of PMT

There is a great deal of evidence to show that women become more anti-social during their premenstrual phase. One study of women prisoners, for example, showed that 49 per cent had committed their crimes during this time. Another study showed that 52 per cent of admissions for accidents in four London teaching hospitals occurred in women during the few days before menstruation. Other studies show that during this time women are also more likely to become violent with husbands and children, get drunk and attempt suicide. In other words, one might say that during their premenstrual phase women are more likely to start behaving like men since men generally commit more crimes, get drunk more often and display violence more frequently.

Obviously this is disturbing for the woman who finds herself being rather more wild than usual. Unfortunately that is rarely the reason why the statistics are produced. More often they are used to prove that women are unreliable by virtue of their menstrual cycle. The fact that men indulge in far more extreme and anti-social behaviour without benefit of a menstrual cycle is usually overlooked.

There is a theory presented by Peter Redgrove and Penelope Shuttle in their book *The Wise Wound* that menstruation is the time in a woman's cycle when she becomes less inhibited and more prepared to speak the truth about her life. They argue that this is the time when all the frustrations and resentments which are repressed during the rest of the cycle rise to the surface. It's an interesting theory but difficult to prove. We do know, however, that stress effects the severity of premenstrual symptoms. If a woman is involved in something very interesting and exciting, her premenstrual symptoms will vanish for a time; if she is in a very difficult and upsetting situation they will be much worse than usual. So it may be that the premenstrual state simply creates a heightened awareness of what is going on in life and magnifies the mood. Since most women don't lead especially fulfilling lives the mood reflected is usually bad.

There are a few compensations to the premenstrual phase. One study found that among married women 60 per cent found they felt sexier just before menstruation. Again, this could be explained as part of the heightened awareness which occurs at this time. It certainly runs counter to the popular belief that women feel sexiest at the time of ovulation in mid-cycle when they are most likely to conceive. Women also find this is a time when they dream more and one woman I talked to felt she became psychic:

It definitely happens, too often to be coincidence. It may not occur to a lot of people I suppose but I've always been interested in things like that so I notice it. I think you're much stronger as a person during menstruation. You do definitely become more aggressive.

PMT and the Family

If a woman suffers from PMT, it inevitably has an effect on her family. The effect was probably less in the days of large families when there were a number of adults to help with children. Today we live in the smallest possible family unit which means that the moods of the wife and mother become magnified and strongly influence the rest of the family. Small children are especially sensitive to their mother's mood and may only be able to adjust by developing coughs or vomiting or crying endlessly, none of which improves the mother's temper. One study found that in a sample of mother's taking their child to the doctor's surgery 54 per cent were in their premenstrual phase. So if you have a small child who seems to go through frequent bad patches, it is worth noting down the coughs and colds or bad days on your menstrual chart to see if there is a pattern.

The most tragic effect of any form of depression or irritability in a mother is battering or non-accidental injury of children. The aggression can be sudden and explosive. Again, any outbursts like this should be noted on your menstrual chart. It is important for you to feel in some kind of control of what is happening so that you can anticipate and work around these moods. There are effective ways of dealing with feelings of anger towards your children. It is so easy to lash out physically but once you recognise that you are prone to do this, move away from the child as soon as you feel your temper snapping. Leave the room if possible and then try one of the following to get all the anger out:

1. Break something, crockery, bottles, jars, etc.
2. Pound the floor, wall, table – anything is better than hitting the child or an animal.
3. Tear up magazines or newspapers or old clothing.

4. Thump a pillow (this is quieter if you're worried about the neighbours).
5. Scream or cry.
6. Skip very fast with a rope.
7. Run up and down a flight of stairs.
8. Stamp your feet.
9. Wash your face with cold water, if necessary, turn on the shower and get in.
10. Slam a door repeatedly.
11. Make a cup of tea or coffee, anything you find calming.
12. Ring a friend or any person you feel you can trust. It is important to talk about how you are feeling.*

These are simply suggestions and it's a matter of trying them out to find out which one you feel comfortable with. Don't give up if the first one doesn't work, you'll probably find one that does.

A mother's premenstrual moods can also upset teenagers but at least it's possible to explain the problem to them so that they understand what's going on. If mother and teenage daughter find that their periods synchronise and they both suffer from PMT, it's probably wise to avoid contact during tension time if humanly possible.

Husbands are inevitably affected by rows and emotional upset at home and may carry it with them into work. The average adult male, however, ought to be able to cope with the situation with patience and understanding once he understands why it is happening.

One curious research finding is that in a partnership women set the body rhythm. Men develop an ovulation temperature chart similar to the one of the woman they are living with. There is a drop in body temperature at mid-cycle followed by a rise after ovulation. This does not occur in men whose partners are on the pill or pregnant, nor in men living alone or with other men.

The worst effects of PMT, of course, are felt by the woman

*These suggestions come from a leaflet produced by the Post-Partum Counselling Service, Vancouver, Canada.

herself. It's a treadwheel. You feel dreadful and you feel guilty about feeling dreadful which makes you feel worse. The guilt at least can be dealt with by simply accepting that PMT occurs for whatever reason and it is *not your fault*.

Causes

Theories about the cause of women's moodiness and unreliability have changed through the years. In fact women are no more unreliable or moody than men. Only 40–50 per cent of women suffer from PMT and of those who do suffer, most would consider the condition an irritating nuisance rather than a major blight. It should also be noted that the drop in energy which women experience just before a period is often compensated for by a period of increased energy at other times in their cycle.

It is important to accept, therefore, that PMT is a *condition* from which women suffer, not a moral blemish which reflects on their abilities as people. It is important to accept this because there are still doctors practising who choose to believe that menstrual problems are all in the mind and a symptom of unstable character. Needless to say, this attitude does not lead to effective treatment of the premenstrual syndrome.

The most popular theory in circulation at the moment is that PMT is caused by a biochemical imbalance. Hormones are chemical messengers which are carried in the blood-stream. They may be directed at a particular organ such as the ovaries or uterus but they can also effect other parts of the body. Hormones also travel to the brain and their effect on mood is very little understood.

The hormone system of the menstrual cycle is very complicated and different doctors have different theories as to which part of it is to blame for PMT. One of the most influential theories is that of simple progesterone deficiency. Yet another is that the trouble is caused not so much by low levels of progesterone as by some imbalance this causes in the system. Other doctors are concerned about another hormone called *prolactin*, a hormone which stimulates the breasts to produce milk.

Hormone theories are attractive because they look simple and straightforward. Unfortunately, no one entirely understands how the whole system works or what relationship it has to the brain, stress and mood. There is a theory that hormones have a general effect on the brain, creating a state of heightened awareness rather than a direct effect on mood. Yet another theory blames the trouble on brain chemistry, claiming it is due to a shortage of vitamin B6 (pyridoxine). All that is really clear is that there is some relationship between menstrual problems and emotional problems though it is not clear which causes which or whether the relationship is pure coincidence.

There is one very important fact to remember. During the time leading up to menstruation, women face low blood sugar levels. If you further reduce these already low levels by skipping meals, dieting or eating junk food and snacks, you will find the symptoms of PMT are much worse than they need be.

Medical Treatments

If your premenstrual symptoms are severe enough to disrupt your life it is worth going to consult your doctor. What treatment s/he prescribes will depend, of course, on what views they hold on the cause of PMT. Some doctors still regard menstrual problems as trivial and not worthy of attention; others are very suspicious of hormonal therapy. As with everything else, it is a question of being persistent until you find a treatment which helps your particular set of symptoms.

Diuretics

These are drugs which are usually given for bloatedness and water retention. They act on the kidneys, increasing the flow of urine. The diuretics prescribed by doctors are strong drugs and there are dangers attached to their use, the chief of which is the risk of losing too much potassium, which is excreted in the urine. Lack of potassium can cause depression and weakness which will make your premenstrual symptoms worse. It is important, therefore, to stick to the doses prescribed by your doctor and to take the drug for only a few days before your period is due. (More natural methods of dealing with water retention are described in the self-help section of this chapter.)

The contraceptive Pill

Many women find that their PMT symptoms are greatly relieved by going on the Pill. Others find that they become much worse. It depends what your symptoms are and which pill you are taking. There are different brands of the Pill and if the one you are taking seems to make your PMT symptoms worse, you should ask your doctor for a different one. It is not a very good idea to start taking the Pill solely to relieve your premenstrual problems. There are hazards connected with long term use of the Pill which are really only worth taking if you decide this is the form of contraception you wish to use.

Progesterone

Many women who suffer from PMT are known to have low levels of progesterone and it therefore seems sensible for them to be given an extra dose. Unfortunately, however, natural progesterone cannot be taken in tablet form because it is destroyed by the digestive system. It therefore has to be taken either as an injection given daily at the time the menstrual problems occur, or as pessaries or suppositories. There are synthetic forms of progesterone called progestogens which can be taken in pill form. These are not identical to progesterone, however, and according to Dr Katharina Dalton who pioneered work on PMT and progesterone therapy, synthetic progestogens have a limited effectiveness as a treatment for PMT and in many cases may even make matters worse.

One progestogen which closely resembles natural progesterone is called *dydrogesterone.* It is marketed under the name *Duphaston* and is a treatment which many women have found very helpful in relieving symptoms. It is cheaper than natural progesterone and easier to take. However, regular and frequent use of synthetic hormones over a long period of time is potentially risky, so it is wise to discuss the use of this treatment and its possible long term and side effects with your doctor before deciding whether you wish to use it.

Bromocriptine

This is a drug which is used to reduce the amount of prolactin in the body. Prolactin, as was mentioned earlier, is the hormone which is most closely connected with the production of breast milk. It is thought that some women suffer from sore breasts, bloatedness and moodiness just before their periods because they have very high levels of prolactin. In these cases *bromocriptine* may be prescribed but it is a powerful drug so it is advisable to take it for only a short time. In large doses it can cause nausea and vomiting so the usual dose is 2.5 mg daily. One final point to remember is that if you are given this treatment you will have a slightly higher risk of becoming pregnant so be sure to use adequate contraception unless you want to have a baby.

Vitamin B6 (pyridoxine)

Vitamin B6 was originally used to help women who suffered from depression as a result of taking the Pill. It was then discovered that it was also a very useful treatment for PMT. Studies carried out mainly at St Thomas's Hospital, London, have found that over two thirds of the women treated for PMT with this vitamin noticed an improvement in their symptoms and between 40 and 45 per cent considered their worst symptoms cured.

Since pyridoxine is a naturally occurring substance you can obtain it from the chemist without a prescription, though it is fairly expensive. Othewise you can ask your doctor to prescribe it for you. For mild symptoms you should take one 20 mg tablet in the morning and another in the evening, starting three days before your symptoms normally start and finishing when your symptoms normally stop.

If your symptoms are more severe and don't respond to this dosage, then double it to take 40 or 50 mg morning and evening. It is not advisable to take more than the 50 mg dose because the acid content will probably upset your stomach. If taken at these dosages the treatment seems to be free of side effects. There haven't been studies of women taking high doses on a long term basis, so it's impossible to say how safe it is if used for a long time but the vitamin is soluble in water so it's thought the body absorbs what it needs and excretes the rest.

Tranquillisers and anti-depressants

If you are suffering from anxiety and stress anyway and it just becomes much worse before your period, then tranquillisers may help for a short time. They will not treat the PMT itself, however, and they may make you feel rather dopey and even less able to cope. If you find life is generally stressful, it is much more constructive to take stock of your life and see if there is anything you can change or adjust to try and make it less stressful. It is possible to become addicted to tranquillisers if you take them for long enough. Anti-depressant drugs are of little use for premenstrual depression since they have to be taken for at least a week before they begin to work.

PMT is not in itself an illness, though it may sometimes feel like one. So it is not really a good thing to take drugs for it unless you feel it is really necessary. There are a number of self-help methods which you can try first, especially if your symptoms are fairly mild.

Self-help

The first thing to do is to make a menstrual chart. This will enable you to check that your symptoms are in fact connected to your periods. It will also show you what the pattern of your cycle is.

Organise your life as far as possible around your symptoms. If you are working, try to ensure you have a lighter work load during the premenstrual period and then catch up later. If you are at home looking after children, try to arrange for friends to help during that time by taking the children off your hands for part of the day or babysitting so that you can get away from the house.

Talk to your family and friends about your symptoms. It is important that both you and they come to terms with the situation. There is no law either human or divine which dictates that people must be constant and consistent in their moods and actions. If you can come to terms with the fact that your moods change at different times in your cycle, you are likely to feel less tense and guilty about it.

Make sure that you eat properly and that you eat nourishing foods. Try to avoid too much greasy or processed food. Eat plenty of fresh vegetables and fruit and remember that wholemeal bread contains more B vitamins than white bread. Above all, eat regularly, don't be tempted to skip meals and if you don't feel up to preparing elaborate meals it is more nourishing to nibble raw carrot, apple or a salad than cakes and biscuits.

If you have problems with bloatedness try to drink less fluids and take less salt. You could also try drinking black coffee and eating such foods as aubergines, cucumber, strawberries, watercress and watermelon, all of which are substances which naturally increase your urine output and help to relieve problems of fluid retention. If you reduce your salt intake it is a good idea to increase the amount of potassium in your diet since salt and potassium work together in the body. Foods such as bananas, oranges and tomatoes are rich in potassium.

Some women find relaxation exercises such as those described for period pains (see Chapter 3) useful for relieving PMT. Others have found that acupuncture or yoga have been helpful. Since stress always makes premenstrual symptoms worse, anything which helps you to feel more relaxed is worth trying.

Chapter Five

Cystitis

Cystitis may strike any woman down at any time. It is a peculiarly painful and embarrassing female condition and probably the most common and least understood of all those I deal with in this book. It has been estimated that nine out of ten women of childbearing age have suffered from it at some time and there are many for whom it has become an agonising blight:

> I had it on and off over a three-year period. It's agonising. I think I used to go to the loo every minute when it was really bad. There was no way you could work or anything. I always had to go into hospital because I always got bleeding. I wasn't married at the time and I didn't know what the infection was so it was terribly embarrassing.

This woman suffered badly. The symptoms of cystitis are such, however, that others who have less severe attacks find the condition socially difficult, especially when on holiday:

> I can remember hitch-hiking to France with a friend when I had it and actually having to get out of the car in desperation because I just had to wee. My poor friend went mad but I just had to. In fact you pass terribly little each time because you want to do it so frequently.

> I just wanted to go to the loo all the time so I was terrified of not being anywhere near a loo and you can imagine what that's like somewhere like Greece where the loos aren't really usable anyway. And it really hurt. It was like a knife twisting in me.

Cystitis is technically an inflammation of the lining of the bladder but it is much more significant than that to the women who suffer from it. It has been blamed for ruined careers and broken marriages and can totally disrupt a couple's sex life. Doctors are unable to explain why some women suffer from it so badly and are unable to offer any guaranteed cure. Indeed, cystitis has been yet another of those conditions which women suffered in silence until they decided to do something about it for themselves.

The woman who has done more than anyone else is Angela Kilmartin, author of *Understanding Cystitis* and *Cystitis – A Complete Self-Help Guide* and founder of the U & I Club (Urinary and Infection) which teaches women how to prevent and manage cystitis attacks. Angela Kilmartin herself was forced to abandon her career as an opera singer as a result of suffering from cystitis and her marriage almost came to an end. Her work on the subject has been of enormous value for thousands of women.

Urinary infections can be divided into three types: urethritis (of the urethra), cystitis (of the bladder) and pyelitis (of the kidneys). These infections are very often connected because an infection travels upwards into the body. Trouble usually starts as urethritis which is an inflammation of the tube (the urethra) which carries urine from the bladder to the outside of the body. In women this tube is only about an inch long and its opening lies very close to the openings of the vagina and the rectum. It is because of this genital geography that women suffer from cystitis so much more than men. It is simply easier for germs to pass from one opening to another.

Infection will normally start in the urethra and feel like a pricking sensation but because the urethra is so short it can take only an hour or so for it to reach the bladder. When this happens, you are likely to feel a pain in the lower abdomen. Infection may then travel up the ureters or tubes leading to the kidneys. If this happens and the kidneys are involved you develop an ache in the back and usually a fever as well. Infection of the kidneys can be dangerous so it is important not to ignore the early symptoms of cystitis in the hope that they will simply go away.

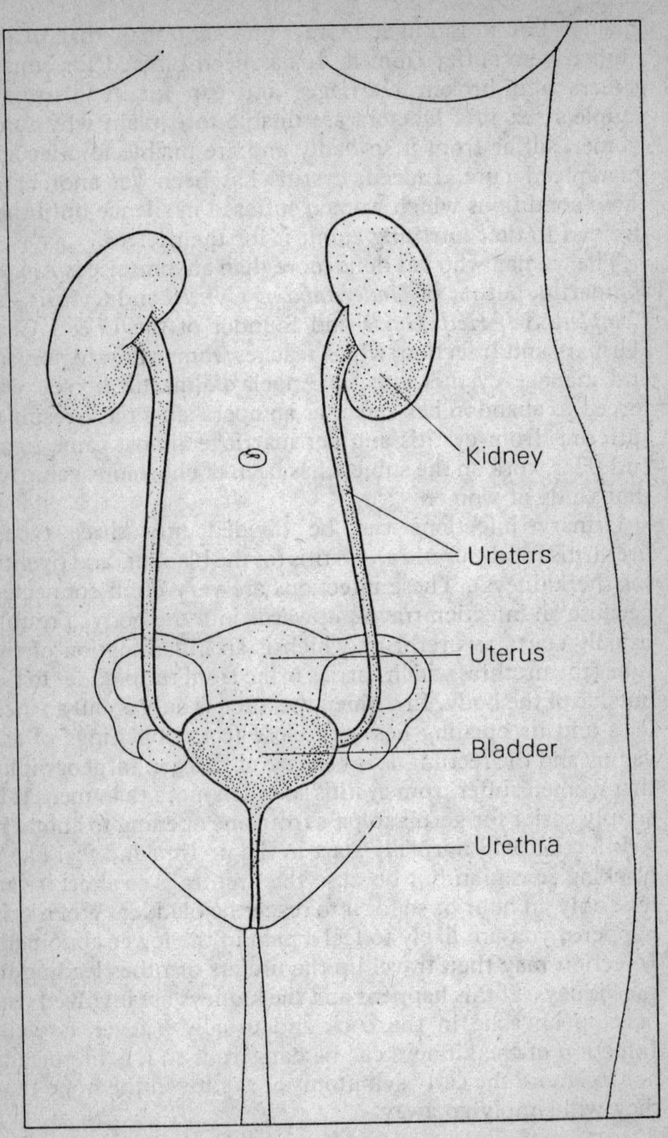
Kidney
Ureters
Uterus
Bladder
Urethra

Causes

The two main causes of cystitis are infection or bruising. Infection usually starts in the urethra and rises to the bladder but it may be present already in the kidneys and bloodstream and descend to the bladder. Bruising usually results from sexual activity and although it seems to present the same symptoms as infection it is really just a swelling of the tissues which become sore and may later become infected.

Cystitis which is caused by bruising is often referred to, somewhat outdatedly, as 'honeymoon cystitis'. This is why many women find the condition so embarrassing:

> I didn't get it treated, very largely because it was embarrassing. Obviously, if I'd started bleeding or if it'd got totally unbearable I *would* have gone to a doctor but as it was I didn't go.

Since infection can pass quickly to the kidneys, it is unwise to ignore an attack of cystitis as this woman did. There are valuable self-help remedies available (which will be described later) and you should have a urine test to establish whether there is an infection present.

The germ which is the main culprit in cases of cystitis is known as E-coli. It normally lives, multiplies and dies in the bowel where it causes no problem. Once outside the bowel, however, it looks for a new breeding ground and will cause trouble if it finds its way into the urine.

Obviously hygiene has an important part to play in preventing the E-coli from moving the short distance between the opening to the rectum and the opening to the urethra. Sex also has an important part to play since any germs lying around the genital area are likely to be thrust forcefully into both vagina and urethra during intercourse. If the urethra is bruised at the same time then trouble is more than likely.

Hygiene in your male partner is also an important factor since you can just as easily be infected with his germs as your own. The foreskin is particularly difficult to clean and can carry any number of bacteria. One woman I talked to found that her boyfriend was the direct cause of her very painful cystitis attacks:

> He was just dirty. He didn't wash. I didn't realise that it was him until after I left him. It just didn't click but the cystitis would clear up and then start again literally every time I had intercourse with this boyfriend.

Having intercourse when your vagina is too dry can cause cracking of the skin of the vagina. This is not only painful, it creates a greater risk of infection since bacteria breed rapidly in even tiny amounts of blood. Any infection of the vagina such as thrush or trichomonas can find its way into the urethra during intercourse and cause problems. And since the antibiotics which are given to cure cystitis very often cause thrush you can easily find yourself on a treadwheel of endless re-infection if you don't watch carefully what's happening.

Cystitis can also be precipitated by sensitivity to the chemicals used in soaps, powders, antiseptic creams and vaginal deodorants. The chemicals which perfume and deodorise toiletries can cause allergic reactions and ironically it is the women most likely to suffer from them that use these things most.

Women who suffer from recurrent cystitis and vaginal infections feel the need to disinfect themselves, not realising that strong antiseptic chemicals irritate an already highly sensitive area and should be avoided like the plague. Nothing is better for personal hygiene than good, old fashioned, pure, clean water.

In fact, anything which disturbs the natural balance of the vagina can also irritate the opening to the urethra and cause trouble. Vaginal cream and foam contraceptives are known to cause problems for some women. It is also known that hormone imbalance, either during the menopause or in women suffering from premenstrual syndrome can precipitate cystitis. This is because hormones control the acid/alkaline balance in the vagina and may produce unhealthy mucus which infects the urethra. In the same way the Pill may predispose some women to cystitis attacks although it may equally prevent them in others. The same situation occurs with pregnancy which triggers chronic urinary infections in some women and, whilst pregnancy lasts, completely clears them up for others.

Other causes of cystitis arise not so much from infection which ascends through the urethra as from problems within the urinary system itself. The most common of these is something called a refluxing ureter. This means that there is a fault in the valve at the top opening to the bladder so that the valve closes before all the urine has passed through the bladder. The remaining urine is pushed back up the ureter towards the kidney where it becomes stale and an ideal breeding ground for bacteria. This is a condition found most frequently in children and usually corrects itself by the age of eight. If it continues after that age then an operation is usually recommended. There are other kidney conditions and infections which predispose women to cystitis but they are not very common. The more usual cause is ascending infections.

No one can really explain why some women never suffer from cystitis and others suffer endlessly. It seems that some women just have more sensitive skins or are more susceptible to infection than others. If you are one of the unlucky ones, however, there is a great deal you can do to help yourself if you get an attack, or more important, prevent attacks from occurring.

Treatment

As soon as you notice the first symptoms follow Angela Kilmartin's advice for managing the attack:

1. Drink a pint of water.
2. Follow this by drinking half a pint of liquid every twenty minutes. Weak tea, diluted fruit squash or plain water are best, *not* concentrated juices.
3. Take a level teaspoon of bicarbonate of soda mixed in water or jam. This makes the urine less acid and helps to stop it from burning. Repeat this dose on the hour every hour for three or four hours. If you have problems with heart trouble

or blood pressure, consult your doctor before taking bicarbonate of soda.

All this is intended to flush out the bladder and you will find that within thirty or forty minutes of starting you will begin to go to the toilet more frequently. It may sting at first but this will go away as more water passes through the bladder.

4. Drink black coffee on the hour every hour for three hours to encourage urination. Do *not* drink alcohol.
5. Make yourself as comfortable as possible. Fill two hot water bottles and settle down with one wrapped carefully between your legs so that both the urethal and vaginal openings have this heat directly on them. The effect of this is to make the skin feel hotter than the urine which reduces the sensation of burning. Place the second hot water bottle against your back.
6. Every time you pass water, no matter how little, wash yourself gently with warm, moist cotton wool and dab yourself dry. Or, alternatively, carefully pour a jug of water at blood heat from the top of the pubis as you sit on the loo. The water trickles down over the vulva and dilutes the urine, then rinses afterwards.

Three hours after starting this treatment the attack will have abated considerably or it will have gone altogether. If it has simply abated then get yourself to the doctor as soon as possible. The doctor will probably want a sample of urine to test, especially if you suffer from recurrent attacks of cystitis, so be prepared either to take one with you or produce one once you get there.

Ideally cystitis should not be treated until a culture growth has been made from a urine sample. This will determine which bacteria is responsible so that the correct drug can be given. Unfortunately this process takes about two and a half days and in the meantime the infection is likely to reach the kidneys and you will be really ill. In practise, therefore, most doctors prescribe antibiotics somewhat haphazardly. For many women this will probably be sufficient and the infection will clear up. For others it will be of little use and simply the beginning of recurrent attacks of cystitis, as this woman found:

> I first noticed it when I was about fourteen. I got this weird prickling sensation every time I passed urine. It worried me because it was very painful. When I was at school it was really inconvenient as well because I had to keep being excused to go to the loo. So I went to see the doctor – my family GP and of course he told my Mum, so I got a right telling off because I didn't tell her. It happened again after I left home when I was sixteen. The doctor called it 'honeymoon cystitis' whatever that might be. He gave me some tablets, I don't remember what they were now. It seemed to me that I'd take a course of tablets and I'd be all right for a bit and then it'd flare up again and I'd be back on the tablets again. I got really fed up with taking tablets. I was on them about a year altogether.

This pattern of recurrence may occur because the antibiotic causes thrush which re-infects the urethra or it may be that you are being prescribed the wrong antibiotic, or it may be that you require further specialist investigations to find out what is causing the attacks.

The specialist you should be referred to is a urologist. S/he is the expert on renal organs and the urinary system. S/he will want a sample of urine for tests and will usually give you an X-ray called an IVP. This consists of injecting dye into a vein which shows up well on X-ray. As the dye passes through your kidneys, ureters and bladder, several pictures are taken which will tell the urologist if there is anything unusual in your system.

If your urine test and X-ray are normal, you're likely to be back on antibiotics until you are sent for the next investigation which is called a cystoscopy. This is a minor operation, usually done under a general anaesthetic with an instrument called a cystoscope. Using this the urologist can look into your bladder and see whether there are scars and thickened skin. If there is, s/he may burn away the infected skin. Unfortunately, this is unlikely to be very effective. What is often more effective, though only for a short while, is the dilation of the urethra. This may have been damaged by previous attacks and have narrowed so that urine is not being flushed out very effectively and is harbouring germs. The conditions which produced the damage in the first place still exist, however, and symptoms are likely to recur.

If, after all this, you find that you *still* suffer from recurrent attacks of cystitis, then you should have a thorough gynaecological examination. Many of the causes of recurrent cystitis lie in your reproductive organs and a urologist won't discover those.

All these medical investigations take time and patience but meanwhile you can be helping yourself by following the self-help procedures already outlined and by doing your own detective work. Make a note of each attack and the circumstances connected to it, including the time in the menstrual cycle, length of time since last attack, connection with sex, contraceptive use, use of any toiletries, in fact anything that seems remotely relevant. As Angela Kilmartin writes:

> Eliminate all thoughts of CURE from your mind. There isn't a cure and never will be because cystitis is only a symptom. What you have to do first of all is to think for yourself and for your doctor what might be causing the recurrent attacks.

Once you are satisfied that medical examination proves you have nothing organically wrong with you, and you hopefully have some idea of what *is* causing your attacks, then you can concentrate on prevention.

Prevention

1. *Diet:* Drink plenty of plain water as often as possible. Avoid alcohol completely and cut down on coffee and tea (coffee is helpful only when an attack has already started as part of treatment). These excite the kidneys and bladder

which need to be kept calm. Avoid hot curries and spicy food wherever possible, also strawberries and citrus fruit which are acidic and irritate the bladder.

2. *Hygiene:* E-coli is a common germ which is responsible for much cystitis. It lives in the bowel and can easily contaminate the urethra. After bowel movements *always* wipe your bottom from front to back to avoid contamination. If you suffer from recurrent attacks of cystitis, *wash* your perineum from front to back each time you have a bowel movement, but make sure that you wash your hands first. *Never* use antiseptic tissues or any form of disinfectant, they will cause irritation.

3. *Sex:* Genital skin is highly sensitive, and prolonged, vigorous and frequent intercourse can make you sore and bruised. The anser is not celibacy but care. *Before* you have intercourse empty your bladder, wash your hands and then wash your perineum with plain water to ensure that any lurking germs are washed away. This is not very romantic but then neither is an attack of cystitis. *After* intercourse empty your bladder again and then pour cool water from a bottle or jug over your perineum to reduce inflammation and pat yourself dry with a clean towel.

Ensure that your partner has washed his hands and penis before intercourse. He can just as easily infect you with his germs as with your own. Don't permit penetration if you are too dry. You can always use KY jelly to improve lubrication and it is important to avoid bruising.

4. If you feel the slightest twinge of an attack start the self-help procedure immediately. This has been found so helpful by so many women it should be handed out by all GPs and all clinics.

5. If you suffer from recurrent attacks of cystitis, buy yourself a copy of *Cystitis, A Complete Self-Help Guide* by Angela Kilmartin which covers ever aspect of this subject in far more detail than you will find here and has been a great help and comfort to thousands of sufferers.

Chapter Six

Thrush and Other Itches

Vaginal infections itch. They may be extremely painful, they may produce a foul discharge, but above all else, they itch intolerably:

> I had no idea what it was, absolutely no idea. I thought I'd got some ghastly rash. It lasted about three weeks. The itching was terrible; I couldn't sleep at night, it was hot weather, I remember.

This woman was, in fact, suffering from an attack of thrush, but it could as easily have been another vaginal infection. Since some infections are more serious than others, this is one area where an examination is important to determine exactly what infection you have. Unfortunately, it is also an area where the average GP is very reluctant to examine:

> One thing I found, which is very, very bad is that so few GPs will examine you. They won't examine you and take a swab because they don't want to dirty their surgery or whatever; they just *don't* want to examine you. I've never had a GP that's examined me for thrush or taken a swab.

Doctors I talked to agreed that this was often the case. As one explained to me:

> That's why drug companies come round with the all-purpose pill, the all-purpose pessary or the all-purpose cream. You don't have to think, you just prescribe it. The chances are that it'll sort out all the infective causes but the trouble is that it won't actually catch the erosions and it

won't catch the carcinomas either, which, of course, are the nasty ones. I would normally examine women who came with these problems, take a swab, maybe actually take a smear as well. The other doctor is working on probabilities. Apart from saying, 'I'm too lazy to bother,' he's saying, 'I know that something like 95 per cent of the women with these symptoms will get better with this all-purpose drug.' So he's taking a calculated risk that he's going to miss something in, say 5 per cent of his patients. But I would say that the average woman who comes to me with this problem feels better going out of the room knowing she's been properly checked rather than just given something. I mean there's no point in quoting statistics to patients because the problem is personal.

In fact no drugs are completely harmless, they are all powerful chemicals which is why they are effective. We should not be expected to take unnecessary drugs when it is a relatively simple matter for the doctor to diagnose which vaginal infection we are suffering. If your GP refuses to examine you or wants to prescribe without examining you then you should ask him or her why. If you find his or her answer unsatisfactory, then you can either change your GP, go to a Well-Woman Clinic, go to a Special Clinic or try and consult a gynaecologist privately.

It has been suggested that in some cases both vaginal discharges and cystitis may be caused by food allergies which inflame the mucus membranes. The foods most often implicated are dairy produce such as milk, cheese and butter. If you have recurrent problems it is worth changing your diet to avoid these products and see if this has any effect.

Thrush

Thrush is a yeast or fungus infection. It causes severe itching, inflammation and soreness and there are white spots in and around the vagina. Intercourse is usually painful and should be avoided as your partner may catch the thrush and re-infect you. Thrush doesn't always produce a discharge but when it does the discharge is thick and white like cottage cheese and smells yeasty like baking bread. This woman's experience is fairly typical:

> There was a bit of a discharge. I don't think I was looking for a discharge at the time though, I was just aware of being red, redder than normal. I had a look with a mirror and it was a bit spotty. The doctor did ask if my husband had it and I said that he was a bit sore from time to time. So it turned out that we'd been re-infecting each other all the time.

The particular yeast fungus responsible for thrush is called *candida albicans* or *monilia*. It normally lives in harmless numbers in the vagina and rectum, for like all warm, wet places, our vaginas are teeming with microscopic life. Whole colonies of different bacteria and fungus live and die quite harmlessly there. They are kept in control by the normal acid-alkaline balance of the vagina and provided nothing happens to disturb their environment we live quite happily in harmony with them.

It is when the chemical balance of the vagina changes that we are likely to experience problems. Because if the balance changes then some colonies will be wiped out and others will spread and grow out of all proportion. This is what happens in the case of thrush. Candida prefers a mildly acidic environment and normally the vagina is too strongly acidic to allow it to do more than survive.

There are a number of conditions which can alter the delicate chemical balance of the vagina. Hormonal changes can produce there an ideal environment for thrush. Many women find that they are particularly vulnerable just before, during, or just after their period. Others develop persistent thrush when they start taking the Pill. If this happens to you it would be sensible either to change your brand of Pill or to come off the Pill altogether and use a different contraceptive. Pregnancy is another time when women are very susceptible.

Thrush during pregnancy should be cleared up as soon as possible since your baby is likely to develop it in its mouth (another warm, wet place) if it is present in the vagina at birth.

This is not particularly serious but should be avoided if possible.

Thrush flares up during these times of hormonal change because there is more sugar in the vagina and the yeast, like all yeasts, loves sugar. For the same reason, thrush is a side effect of diabetes. Elderly women who develop thrush should always have a urine check because it can be the first sign of diabetes.

Another major cause of thrush is antibiotics which may be taken for a throat or chest infection, or for cystitis. Antibiotics kill bacteria but they do so quite indiscriminately. So whilst the antibiotic is attacking the bacteria which make you ill, it is also killing off the bacteria in your vagina which keep the candida population under control and thrush results.

Bacteria in the vagina can also be killed by any of a number of chemical substances which are introduced into the vagina such as deodorants, bubble bath or perfumed soaps. These may cause severe irritation and expose you to the risk of infection.

Treatment

Medical treatment usually consists of nystatin pessaries which are rather messy but usually effective. Sometimes nystatin in pill form is prescribed but should only be taken if absolutely necessary since it kills off fungi of other kinds in the body and may occasionally make you feel nauseous.

One effective treatment which is often used for very stubborn cases of thrush is to paint the cervix, vagina and vulva with gentian violet. This is rather messy and makes you an interesting colour, so it's a good idea to wear a sanitary pad during treatment to stop your clothes turning purple.

Self-help

These treatments can be useful but they need to be started as soon as you feel the slightest itch because they are much less effective once the yeast infection really takes hold. The most popular self-help remedy for thrush is natural yoghurt. This is not the yoghurt that you buy at your local supermarket which is dead yoghurt, but the live yoghurt which you can buy in a health food shop.

Live yoghurt contains bacteria which help to keep yeast under control which is why this remedy is thought to work, though there has been no research into it. It is probably most effective as a treatment if it is inserted into the vagina. This can be done by first warming the yoghurt to hand temperature but no warmer. If you make it too hot, you will kill the bacteria. Next fill a tampon applicator with yoghurt, keeping the tampon in the end so that is doesn't run out. Insert the yoghurt and the tampon slowly into your vagina. This procedure should be repeated every few hours. An alternative method is one described by one of the women I spoke to:

> Live yoghurt clears it up a treat. I lie on my back with my feet in the air and just pour it in, just a cupful of it. I put the whole cupful in and then lie with my legs straight up on the wall and my head raised slightly. I just lie there and read a book for about half an hour. It's a bit messy but I prefer to do it that way, and it works.

Some women also eat yoghurt, as a treatment, but this has a more gradual effect over a period of time.

Another self-help remedy worth trying is to have a bath with some cider vinegar in it, just water and vinegar of course, no soap. Make sure that the vinegar water gets into your vagina. Vinegar is acidic and this helps to restore the proper acid balance of the vagina.

As with cystitis, the important thing is to catch the infection in time and act quickly. If you allow the yeast to develop it can become the very devil to get rid of. If you find that you are prone to attacks of thrush then concentrate on prevention.

Prevention

Infections have the best chance of thriving when you are most run down and tired and your body can offer least resistance. A healthy diet, sensible exercise, proper sleep and a relaxed mind are the best general preventative medicine. In addition, if you suffer from recurring attacks of thrush you can help yourself by following a few basic rules:

1. Don't put anything in your vagina that you wouldn't put in your mouth.
2. Keep the area round your vagina dry and airy.
3. Wear pure cotton pants or no pants. Nylon creates heat and doesn't allow the skin to breathe properly. Avoid wearing tights and tight trousers for the same reason.
4. Wash your vulva and rectum regularly and pat dry. Avoid irritating sprays, perfumed soaps and bubble bath.
5. Ensure that your sexual partner washes carefully before making love.
6. Don't resume sexual intercourse too soon after an attack of thrush. Wait until the soreness has gone.
7. Check the contraceptive you are using. Some women are constantly re-infected because they have a coil. Many women develop thrush because they are on the Pill. Chemical foams can cause irritation.
8. Check that your sexual partner doesn't have thrush. It's possible that you may be constantly re-infecting each other. If he does have thrush he will probably notice itching and irritation of his penis as well as redness and soreness. He may also have a discharge, but not necessarily. He may have no symptons, in which case he should go to be checked if you suffer from recurring attacks.

Thrush doesn't attack or harm your uturus or Fallopian tubes and will not affect your fertility.

Non-Specific Vaginitis

In medical jargon the term 'itis' at the end of a word means 'inflammation of' and in the case of vaginitis it's inflammation of the vagina. Non-specific means that the bug causing the infection is unknown though in fact lab tests can usually sort out which one it is.

The symptoms are a discharge which may be white, yellow or grey-green and it may have a foul smell. Sometimes there are also symptoms like cystitis (see Chapter 5), pain in the vagina after intercourse and, of course, the inevitable itching.

It is important to have a culture taken in order to find out whether the infection is bacterial or viral. Bacterial vaginitis may be transmitted by sexual intimacy or it may arise spontaneously. If the discharge is bacterial you may be prescribed cream or pessaries to clear up the infection. If no bacteria are found you will probably be given an antibiotic. It is a good idea for your partner(s) to be checked as well, just in case they are also infected.

Trichomoniasis

Trichomonas (trick-o-moan-as) vaginitis is an infection caused by a one-celled parasite called a trichomonad.

Infection is usually transmitted sexually but the parasite can live for a few hours outside the body in puddles of water or moist objects. So it is possible to contract it from damp towels, bathing suits, flannels, underwear or toilet seats. In men the infection rarely has any symptoms which means that they are more often carriers rather than sufferers. Women usually do have symptoms though sometimes they are so slight that they may be ignored. It is thought that between 30 and 40 per cent of women who have trichomoniasis also have gonorrhoea so it is important to have it diagnosed and treated properly.

The symptoms of trichomoniasis are a frothy, thin vaginal discharge which is yellowish-green or grey in colour and has a foul smell. Women also complain of cystitis-like symptoms (see Chapter 5) and indeed trichomonas can cause urinary infection. The infernal itch may be on the thighs as well as the vulva and you are likely to be rather sore.

Treatment

Trichomoniasis is usually treated with a drug called Flagyl (metronidazole). Flagyl is a very powerful drug and the American Food and Drug Administration have approved an information leaflet for American doctors that accompanies each package of the drug. It contains the warning that Flagyl has been shown to be cancer-producing in mice and possibly in rats. It recommends that a white blood cell test should ideally be taken both before and after treatment because Flagyl may temporarily decrease the body's ability to produce white cells (leukocytes). It is the white blood cells which fight infection so it can be quite dangerous to have too few of them. It is especially important to have a test before beginning a second course of Flagyl.

At the moment these warnings are issued only in America and medical opinion in Britain is that the drug is relatively safe. It may be that many British doctors are not aware of the American research for Flagyl tends to be prescribed rather liberally. There is, indeed, an all-purpose pack consisting of Flagyl for trichomoniasis and nystatin for thrush which many GPs will prescribe for any vaginal discharge on the basis that if one doesn't cure it the other one will, since most vaginal discharges are either thrush or trichomoniasis. Not entirely scientific, but it saves time. Unfortunately Flagyl can sometimes *cause* thrush, apart from its other disadvantages, so you may well be on a merry-go-round if you start such treatment.

If you happen to have a doctor who won't examine you and prescribes one of these all-purpose packs you would be well advised to visit a Special Clinic where swabs will be taken and the infection properly diagnosed. Flagyl is an extremely efficient drug for clearing up trichomoniasis but it should be taken with caution and you need to be sure not only that the condition has been properly diagnosed but that gonorrhoea is not present as well.

If you are prescribed Flagyl, you should remember the following:

1. Flagyl should not be taken if you have peptic ulcers, another infection elsewhere in the body, a history of blood diseases or a disease of the central nervous system.
2. Flagyl should be avoided if possible if you are pregnant or breast feeding.
3. Side effects of Flagyl may include nausea, dizziness, cramps, diarrhoea, gastric upsets, furring of the tongue and a bad taste in the mouth. It can cause blood disorders; you may develop thrush as a result of taking it and some women find it causes depression or sleepiness.
4. While taking Flagyl you must avoid alcohol as the combination will almost certainly produce some side effects.

5. Wait at least four to six weeks after treatment before starting a second course of treatment.
6. The manufacturers recommend taking a blood test after treatment and, with a repeat course, blood should be tested before, during and afterwards.
7. Your regular partner(s) should be treated as well to avoid the ping-pong of re-infection.
8. You should have no sex during treatment.

There are vaginal pessaries and vaginal gels which can provide adequate treatment but may not be as effective as Flagyl. Exposure to the air destroys the trichomonas parasites so wearing loose cotton clothing, cotton pants or no pants at all, avoiding chemicals in toiletries and having regular baths should help to prevent recurrences of infection.

One woman I talked to who developed trichomonas treated it effectively by using garlic which is known as 'nature's antibiotic'. With this treatment you obviously smell rather strongly for a while but it offers a possible alternative to drugs:

> I didn't want to take Flagyl because I was pregnant and even when I'm not I avoid drugs as far as possible. Luckily a friend knows a lot about alternative treatments and as soon as I had a positive diagnosis she recommended the garlic. I used a clove of garlic as a pessary and I used calendula as an ointment for swabbing my vulva. I kept the clove in place with a piece of natural sponge and used a fresh clove each morning and thoroughly rinsed the sponge. Calendula is a common garden plant. I used a handful of leaves to one pint of water simmered for twenty minutes. I used it for three days and then made a fresh solution. I also stopped wearing pants and swabbed every time I went to the loo and I took garlic pearls that I got from a health food shop by mouth. When I was checked the infection had gone.

Trichomonas does not attack or harm your uterus or tubes but it may encourage the development of venereal warts. So it is worth keeping an eye open for warts developing around the entrance to your vagina or on your partner's penis. If you see any, seek prompt treatment. The next chapter will deal with this and other venereal diseases.

Chapter Seven

Venereal Diseases

Attitudes to venereal disease are rarely well-balanced. We associate it with prostitution, public lavatories and promiscuity, not nice subjects for nice people like you and me. Ignorance breeds fear. To admit to such an infection can seem like proclaiming ourselves to be moral lepers; as one woman told me:

> It's something that really I don't think I've ever discussed with anybody because I felt so guilty about it and so sort of dirty.

Young women suffer agonies of anxiety over a simple case of thrush because it just might be ... and women who suspect their partner's fidelity feel both humiliation and betrayal:

> I was paranoid about it because he actually did give me gonorrhoea. He met me from work one day and he said, 'There's something wrong with me, I'm all sort of swollen and sore, I think I'd better go to the doctor,' and my heart sank and I thought, 'Oh, God, I don't believe it,' because I knew that if he had it would mean that it was going to come out that he'd been screwing around and I didn't want to know. I was so madly in love with him I felt I'd rather ignore it, I'd rather not know. Anyway he had it so I went down to the Special Clinic and they did tests. Then they called me in and said, 'You've got gonorrhoea,' and I just dissolved, I was in hysterics. The nurses were lovely but I said, 'You don't understand, it's my fiance, we were going to get married,' and she said, 'I'm sorry. I'm afraid we see so much of it.'

And so it goes. It's not an easy subject to treat objectively. Indeed, of all aspects of our sexuality, this is probably the most guilt inducing. Admitting secrets to a strange doctor is far from easy.

Of course sex is less secretive and furtive than it used to be but attitudes change a great deal more slowly than many of us would like to believe. Ideally venereal disease should be treated much like any other disease, without embarrassment, and hopefully this will happen in time. At the moment Special Clinics in hospitals are often hidden away in dark basements where there can only be an air of furtiveness:

> I went for a check at a clinic once. They're very impersonal, you just get a card and a number. You have to sit in a waiting room and they call the number. They're usually down a side street but you don't have to let it make you feel seedy. I suppose they do it like that because if it was obvious where you're going an awful lot of people probably would never go. I think youngsters especially should know about it. It's one of those things you just don't talk about.

Sometimes staff in Special Clinics seem to have an over-exaggerated concern to protect what they suspect will be your natural sense of shame at being there. They are, however, considerably less patronising on the whole than many gynaecologists who deal with unwanted pregnancies.

'Venereal disease' is, in fact a legal term. The medical term is 'sexually transmitted diseases'. Correctly, VD refers to only three conditions, gonorrhoea, syphilis and chancroid. These were the three diseases of most public concern in 1917 when the Veneral Diseases Act was passed. Chancroid, a so-called tropical venereal disease, was very common at that time. Today it is very rare. Instead, the majority of patients attending Special Clinics suffer from a wide variety of other conditions which are sexually transmitted.

In practice the only real difference between venereal disease and sexually transmitted disease is legal not medical. If you offer to treat gonorrhoea and syphilis without being medically qualified you can be put in prison, for example, and these diseases can be claimed as grounds for divorce, and be relevant in cases of rape. But since the very term VD carries with it so many connotations of guilt and immorality, it is to be hoped that in time the term will be dropped.

Unfortunately the incidence of sexually transmitted diseases is growing, especially amongst young people. The areas where it is really taking off are the non-specific infections and genital herpes though there is also a rise in the incidence of gonorrhoea. The spread of infection in Britain, however, is nothing like as dramatic as it is in America. This is chiefly because Britain has such a highly organised and efficient free clinic system.

There are a number of reasons why sexually transmitted diseases are on the increase. Attitudes towards most sexual activities are more permissive. Unfortunately, however, the flood of information on how, when and where to do it has not been matched by sensible information on how to either avoid or cope with the consequences of doing it. This leaves young people particularly in a very vulnerable situation.

Travel has always been a major factor in the spread of STD and in recent years there has been an enormous increase in physical mobility. With package tours, group travel and business trips, the world has become the proverbial village. People let their hair down when they're away from home and in doing so risk contracting disease and carrying it back with them. And when continents are involved instead of counties, tracing and treating contacts from such liaisons is a major headache.

A much more worrying factor is the increasing resistance to antibiotics of some of the bacteria which cause STD. This trend has been most marked with gonorrhoea, and most particularly in the Far East, South East Asia (the result of the Vietnam war) and the western states of the USA. The problem is that bacteria are living organisms and just as rats will become resistant to poison if they survive taking a dose, so bacteria will develop resistance to penicillin if the whole colony is not killed. For this reason, it is vital to take the full course that is prescribed and to be fully checked afterwards to ensure that none of the bacteria have managed to survive.

Unfortunately, this doesn't happen in third world countries where antibiotics are often sold from a market stall, literally by the handful, according to what you can afford, which usually isn't much. Because too little penicillin is taken, therefore, some bacteria survive which are then spread round the population and eventually travel to other countries.

There are not, so far, any strains which are resistant to all antibiotics, but the trend is potentially very serious. Most clinics in England screen all cases of gonorrhoea for penicillin resistance.

The general view of STD throughout history has been that it is a tragedy for men to contract disease, but criminal for women. Indeed, in the Contagious Diseases Act of 1864, provision was made for the arrest of women suspected of spreading infection and their compulsory examination and detention. Considerable agitation from women's groups led to the repeal of the act in 1886. But the idea that women were chiefly responsible for the spread of infection proved a persistent one. It is, after all, a view which adheres closely to the dual standard of sexual morality which is only now showing signs of crumbling.

Special Clinics

The estimated population of the United Kingdom is fifty-six million people. This population is served by 230 clinics for STD; 187 are in England, 18 in Scotland, 14 in Wales and 11 in Northern Ireland. These clinics may be called Special Clinics, VD Clinics or Genito-Urinary Departments. All residents of the UK have free access to the clinics, can attend of their own free will and free of charge.

The social importance of such clinics cannot be overestimated. When it was discovered that penicillin would treat syphilis in the 1950s it was decided in America to disband the special clinics and contact tracing, give all doctors penicillin and thus solve the problem of STD and save money at a stroke. The result was that in three years there was a 300 per cent increase in the incidence of syphilis over all and in California the increase was 680 per cent. Clinic facilities had to be resurrected very swiftly.

You do not need to have a letter from your GP to attend a Special Clinic. You may, of course, choose to see your GP first, but s/he is likely to refer you if s/he suspects you have a STD. This is because the Special Clinic has the right facilities for speedy diagnosis and treatment:

> I went to this clinic down a back street. They're always in backstreets, always in basements and pretty seedy. The waiting room was always crowded, it just wasn't well done. But they never made you feel embarrassed and they never made you feel an outcast. They're extremely good and very careful. You have a lot of tests done and it takes a long time. I've always felt they're so much more efficient and caring that I wouldn't go to a GP and ask a GP to do it because they just don't go to the same trouble.

Clinics vary, of course, and some can seem very impersonal, but that is true of all clinics. Some of them are only open part-time during the week, so it is worth checking times by telephoning first. You will find the name of your local clinic by looking in the telephone book under 'Venereal Disease'. For a recorded tape message on symptons you can ring 01-2146-8072.

Treatment of STD is always given in the strictest confidence. When you arrive at the clinic you will probably be asked to give your name and address and the name of your GP. You will not be asked to show your NHS card, so you could give a false name if you wish. If you do give a false name, make a note somewhere what name you used as it can cause endless complications if you forget! There is no compulsion to give your address and you can refuse. Alternatively, you can ask that no correspondence be sent to your address and that will be honoured.

You will next be given a card and a number. Some clinics will call you out by name to see the doctor, others will use your number. Being called by number can seem a bit like being in prison and many clinics are trying to remove that atmosphere of shame and secrecy but it varies from area to area. It is also worth noting that there are a number of female venereologists and if you especially wish to see one you should ask. It may mean making an appointment on a different day if a woman doctor doesn't happen to be on duty, but most clinics will respect your wishes.

When you see the doctor s/he will want to know what your symptoms are, if any, and will then take down your personal and medical history. S/he will want to know when you last had intercourse and how many partners you have had in the last three months because that's the incubation period for syphilis. You are also likely to be asked about contraception since some drugs mustn't be taken early in pregnancy. It is also useful for the doctor to know if sheaths have been used. Sheaths don't offer complete protection, but they do offer some. You might be asked in addition if you have had oral or anal sex.

Obviously it's important to tell the doctor if you are allergic to any antibiotics. It is equally important to tell him or her if you have had antibiotics recently since that can make a difference to the lab results which needs to be allowed for.

Following your interview you will be taken to a consulting room, asked to undress from the waist down and examined. The examination is very thorough and a number of tests are done. These include the taking of a cervical smear, swabs from the vagina and cervix, a pelvic examination and a blood test and urine test. Doctors prefer you not to have urinated for at least two hours before giving a urine sample.

After this you will be asked to wait for the first test results which will be done immediately in the lab. These usually take about fifteen minutes. If the tests are positive you will be treated immediately and there will be no prescription charge. If you are given treatment make sure that you complete the whole course as prescribed and remain celibate until you are told you are free of infection by the clinic.

If your first tests show no infection, you will be asked to return to the clinic for the results of the more extensive culture tests. It is *vital* that you return for these results. If you have gone to the clinic because you are a contact and no infection is found, you may still be asked to take treatment, especially if your partner has a non-specific infection.

Ideally your partner should tell you what infection he has given you, though not all men do. The contact slip will not tell you, it will only give a code. This is to preserve confidentiality. If your partner hasn't been open with you, the doctor may then be in the difficult situation of asking you to take treatment without being able to explain what for.

In women non-specific discharges are not always easy to sort out from normal discharges and if your partner has been found to have a non-specific infection it is probable that he has passed it on to you, even if the clinic cannot definitely prove it. This is why you will be offered antibiotics 'just in case' you have the infection. If you object to this your only real alternative is to wait until he is cured and then sleep with him again and see if he is re-infected. It's a difficult decision to take but only you can balance the risks for yourself.

The testing at the clinics are so thorough because very often a number of infections occur together and the clinic needs to ensure that they have all been traced and treated.

Contact tracing

Control of sexually transmitted diseases is in everybody's interests and depends to a great extent on being able to trace and treat both the person who infected you and any people you may have subsequently infected.

You will therefore be asked to contact any sexual partners who may be infected and ask them to attend the clinic. In many clinics you will be given a special contact slip which is a paper with the name, address and telephone number of the clinic and its opening times. You will be asked to talk to your sexual contact(s) and to persuade them to come to the clinic, bringing the contact slip with them. In this way a check can be kept as to whether contacts are turning up for examination. If they don't attend, then a special team of social health workers have the difficult and delicate task of tracing them.

It is important to co-operate with this tracing process even if it places you in a difficult situation, as it might if you're having an extra-marital affair, for example. If you feel unable to tell your partner the truth, you can always suggest you have a urinary infection and he needs to be treated as well. But if you do decide to resort to deception for some reason you should explain to the clinic that you are doing so.

Gonorrhoea

Gonorrhoea is one of the commonest infectious diseases in the world. The World Health Organisation estimates that there are over 250 million people infected with the disease every year and consider it to be completely out of control. Since some of the strains are already virtually penicillin resistent it is vital to have it properly diagnosed and treated.

Gonorrhoea is caused by a bacterium called *gonococci* which thrives in warm, moist places and dies in less than a minute outside the body. It is almost always spread by sexual contact though it is possible to transfer it from discharge on the hands, especially to the eyes. Occasionally, if the mother is infected, the germ is transmitted to the eyes of new born babies. The incubation period is usually two to ten days but can be as long as thirty days.

Unfortunately, as many as 60 per cent of women develop no symptoms at all which means you can harbour and pass on the infection without realising it. It also means that more serious complications can develop because the germs have a chance to breed and travel up from the cervix and through the uterus into the Fallopian tubes.

The minority of women who do develop symptoms complain of vaginal discharge and possibly pain on urination if the urethra has also been infected. Occasionally the rectum also becomes infected by the vaginal discharge which causes anal irritation, discharge and pain when you empty your bowels.

Once the infection spreads to the Fallopian tubes you are likely to feel pain in your lower abdomen, feverish and sometimes sick. These symptoms are often mistaken for appendicitis and can be very dangerous if not dealt with quickly. Inflammation of the Fallopian tubes is called *salpingitis*. It leaves scars and can lead to sterility if the tube is blocked. If the tube is simply narrowed an egg may be fertilised but be unable to travel down the tube to the womb.

This is called an ectopic pregnancy and can be life-endangering (see Chapter 11) It is estimated that about one woman in five who is infected with gonorrhoea develops salpingitis and of these 25 per cent are left with impaired fertility.

The majority of men show symptoms of gonorrhoea in the form of a thick, creamy discharge within a week of being infected. Most women, therefore, first learn that they are infected through being informed by their partner. If this happens it's essential that you go for tests even if you don't have any symptoms. If you develop a discharge yourself which may be trichomoniasis, you should also be screened for gonorrhoea since the two are present together in 50 per cent of cases.

If you suspect that you might have gonorrhoea, go to a Special Clinic immediately, even if your partner has no symptoms. It is not easy to diagnose and you may need to have more than one test done, usually a week apart. Do persevere. If your test is negative and you still feel uneasy, ask for a second test to be done.

Don't wash your vagina or pass urine before the tests are done or you risk washing away the easily available bacteria. 50 per cent of infected women also have an infection in the anus, so an anal swab will probably be taken as well.

It is very important that an accurate diagnosis should be made since different infections require different treatment and the bacteria can develop a resistance to antibiotics. If your partner has been diagnosed as having gonorrhoea you will probably be offered treatment even if your own tests are negative. Discuss this with the doctor if you feel unhappy about it.

Treatment

The normal treatment is a high dose of penicillin injected into the muscle of your buttock or leg. Penicillin works very quickly and effectively when it is given in this way. If you are allergic to penicillin you will be offered an alternative antibiotic in tablet form. If you are given tablets make sure that you finish the whole course or you may encourage the growth of bacteria resistent to antibiotics.

Remember to return to the clinic for tests after treatment so that you can be certain the infection has been cleared. Also ensure that your partner is tested and treated if necessary so the re-infection doesn't occur.

Sometimes treatment for gonorrhoea can disguise early syphilis without curing it, so it is wise to have a test for syphilis three months after treatment for gonorrhoea.

Syphilis

Syphilis is caused by a tiny, slender, corkscrew-shaped organism called *treponema pallidum* which is capable of living for only a few hours outside the human body. The incidence of syphilis in women has remained steady for some years but it still occurs and must be taken very seriously since its long-term effects include paralysis, heart disease and insanity. Once the bacteria have entered the body the disease goes through four stages.

Primary (early syphilis) The first sign is usually a sore or ulcer called a chancre. This appears anything between one week and three months after you have been infected and usually develops in the place where the bacteria entered the body. In women this is usually on the cervix, vaginal walls or vaginal lips, though it may sometimes appear on the tongue, throat, lips, nipple or finger. The sore looks like a pimple, blister or just an open sore. It is painless, it doesn't itch and it is not tender to touch so it often goes unnoticed, especially in women, where it may be hidden inside the vagina.

The sore occurs as a result of the body fighting to defend itself against the invasion of bacteria. This early stage of syphilis is highly infectious because the sore is full of bacteria which are easily passed to others but, unfortunately, blood tests are negative so it is necessary to examine fluid from the sore to make a diagnosis. If it is left untreated, the sore will heal within one to six weeks. By that time the bacteria have broken through all the defences and invaded every system and organ of the body.

Secondary This stage occurs at any time from a week to six months after the primary sore appears. Because the bacteria are now in the body there are many possible symptoms. You may develop a rash which is symmetrical, coppery-red and does not itch or hurt. Sores may appear in your mouth or throat. You may suffer from swollen glands in the groin, neck and under the chin. Your bones may be affected leading to inflammation and pain. Infection of the scalp may lead to patchy baldness. Or you may have a sore throat, headache and low-grade fever. So many of these symptoms are common to a number of infections that they are easily mis-diagnosed as something else.

At this point you are still infectious and the disease can be spread by any physical contact, like kissing, because any sores are teeming with bacteria which can pass through the pores of the skin. Untreated secondary syphilis tends to come and go with varying degrees of intensity for up to four or five years. The symptoms then disappear but the disease remains active in the body.

Latent Now there is a lull in the battle between the bacteria and the body which may last for as long as thirty years. There are no symptoms and after the first few years of this stage the disease is no longer infectious. It is still in the body, however, and may flare up again.

Late This is the most serious phase of the disease and the reason why it was so feared in the past. Having been latent for many years the bacteria become active again and proceed to attack one of the major organs of the body and cause blindness, serious heart disease or paralysis and insanity. It is very rare indeed for anyone to reach this stage without treatment these days.

Diagnosis of Syphilis

Diagnosing early syphilis is quite difficult so it is important to go to a clinic if you develop any suspicious-looking sores. Don't put any cream or ointment on the sore or you may kill some of the bacteria which are needed to make a diagnosis.

Once the disease has entered the bloodstream, your body will create antibodies to fight it and these will show up in a blood test. So from the secondary stage on, blood tests will reveal the presence of infection.

Treatment
The treatment of syphilis is usually an injection of penicillin into the muscle of the leg or buttock. How much is given will depend on the stage of the disease. It is very important to complete the course and to have at least two follow-up blood tests to be sure you are cured. The first three stages of syphilis can be cured completely by penicillin and the destructive progress of the late stage can be halted.

Congenital Syphilis
One of the nastiest features of syphilis is that it can be passed on by a pregnant woman to her unborn child. Syphilis in a baby can cause defects of the major organs which can be life-threatening and may not show up for years. In the first sixteen weeks of pregnancy the baby is not affected so ideally treatment should be given in the early months. Antenatal clinics screen blood routinely for syphilis at the first appointment, so it is important to attend for that appointment as soon as you think you are pregnant.

Penicillin will stop the disease even if the foetus is affected but it cannot repair any damage already done. So it is especially important to have thorough tests if you suspect you may have caught syphilis while you are pregnant.

Yaws
Yaws is a disease caused by a bacterium very similar to syphilis. It is not a sexually transmitted disease but it gives the same reactions in blood tests as syphilis. It is chiefly a tropical disease and women who have spent their childhood in the tropics may have had yaws without realising it. If this is the case, your blood test may show positive results for syphilis. It's useful to know that there can be false positive results on syphilis tests so that you don't feel too upset if they occur. Special Clinics can usually sort out the situation with further blood tests.

Non-Specific Urethritis
This disease is very much on the increase. In women it rarely

has any symptoms which means they can act as carriers unless they are asked to go to a clinic as a contact:

> So off I went to the Special Clinic with my little label that he'd given me, feeling absolutely ill. I don't remember having any symptoms as all. Still, at least the bloke was honest with me. He'd given me NSU. I tried to find out about it but I couldn't find out much and I've had a phobia about it ever since because you don't have any symptoms as a woman.

In men it causes a discharge from the penis. This discharge is checked by the clinic to see if it is gonorrhoea. If it is non-gonorrhoeal it is called non-specific meaning that the bacterium causing it is unknown.

It has recently been discovered that half of non-specific discharges are caused by minute micro-organisms called *chlamydia trachomatis*. Chalamydia can be grown in the laboratory though not all laboratories in the country have the facilities to grow it since it requires highly specialised techniques. The remaining discharges are still a mystery though venereologists suspect there is a bacterium causing them since they clear up with antibiotics.

It is much more difficult to make a diagnosis with women, so a woman is likely to be offered antibiotics if her male partner has been found to have a non-specific discharge. If a woman has NSU and it is not treated the infection may spread up to her internal organs and cause pelvic inflammatory disease (see Chapter 11). It can also cause conjunctivitis and if the cervix is infected with chlamydia when you are pregnant, the baby may develop an eye infection shortly after it is born.

NSU is normally treated with antibiotics from the tetracycline group. During treatment avoid eating dairy products since they prevent the drug from working effectively. Also avoid alcohol and sex until you have been cleared.

Genital herpes

Herpes is a very common virus. In different forms it causes cold sores, chickenpox and shingles. The *herpes simplex 2* virus causes genital herpes which is a very contagious sexually transmitted disease. Indeed, the incidence of genital herpes has reached epidemic proportions. It is now the fastest-spreading STD in the western world. This is chiefly because, being a virus infection, it's incurable.

Herpes erupts as sores or blisters either around the genital area or inside on the vaginal walls and cervix. The degree of pain felt varies from woman to woman but the sores can be very painful indeed. This is the chief way in which they differ from the ulcers of syphilis. The blisters often burst and leave open sores which are highly contagious and may become infected. If the blisters break out in the urethra, which occasionally happens, you will probably need hospital treatment, since they make it so painful to urinate that the bladder closes up.

Although cold sores on the mouth are caused by a slightly different virus, this form of herpes can easily be transferred to the genitals during oral sex. It is also possible to infect your eyes if you rub them with a finger which has touched a herpes blister. So remember to wash your hands thoroughly after any contact with the sores.

The really nasty thing about genital herpes is that it can't be cured and since it lives in the nerve roots recurrent attacks can occur at any time. The first attack is always the worst. It normally clears within two weeks. Subsequent attacks are less painful but you are just as contagious. This can be nerve-racking, especially if the sores first appear inside the vagina, making it difficult for you to know at any given point whether or not you are infectious to your partner.

There has been some research which suggests that women who have had genital herpes are at risk of developing cervical cancer. The initial research was questioned because it was felt that the two groups of women being studied weren't strictly comparable and so the work is being done again. It is sensible, however, if you have herpes, to make sure that you have a cervical smear taken every six months.

Herpes in Pregnancy

Herpes can be dangerous in pregnancy since the virus can

cross the placenta and damage the foetus, causing miscarriage. If you have open sores at the time of delivery the baby may become infected, suffer from brain damage or die. So it's very important that you inform your midwife or doctor if you have had herpes and become pregnant. Some doctors believe it is wiser to perform a Caesarian section if you have herpes when you go into labour. Again, this is a situation where you must assess the risks for yourself after a hopefully informed discussion.

Treatment

Although there is no effective treatment for herpes, it is wise to go to a clinic because there are many different causes of genital ulcers and you need to have them diagnosed properly. If the sores have become infected they will need treating. Otherwise, the clinic can provide you with painkillers.

To try and alleviate the pain, you should keep your genitals cool and well aired (no nylon pants) and bathe in cool, salt water which will both soothe and clean the sores. Rest as much as possible and avoid sex until the attack has cleared.

At the moment research is being conducted into an anti-virus drug which may be effective as a cure for herpes, but it has not yet been shown to be safe. It does, however, hold out some hope for the future.

Otherwise, there are various folk remedies which may or may not work. Some women claim that fasting clears the symptoms early in an attack, others use heat treatment (a hot bath followed by rest with a hot water bottle between the thighs). Homeopathic cures, which involve vaccination with substances that produce similar blisters, seem to have a reasonable success rate (see Chapter 2).

The space between herpes attacks may be weeks or years, but usually a fresh attack is precipitated by some form of stress. If you are anxious, over-tired, emotionally upset or in any way under par, the virus gets the message and attacks. Of course, simply knowing that you have herpes can make you feel anxious and depressed anyway but nonetheless, the best way to prevent attacks is to try not to worry and to take care of yourself by eating properly, not overworking and avoiding late nights where possible. Over a period of years the herpes virus will eventually burn itself out.

Genital warts

Genital warts are caused by a virus. They are very common and they are infectious. They look much like warts which occur elsewhere and are usually sexually transmitted though they can occasionally be passed from the hands to the genitals. They have a long incubation period, usually two or three months, but sometimes as long as nine months, so it may be difficult to know where you caught them.

Warts are normally red, pink or brownish and tend to grow in a cauliflower-like mass. They occur most often on the vulva, vagina, cervix and around the anus. They seem to like warmth and moisture and spread widely during pregnancy.

Treatment

Warts are usually frozen off at the clinic. This is normally effective and is uncomfortable rather than painful. It may require several treatments. Warts do not recur like herpes but since it isn't possible to know the virus is there until it makes a wart, you may find you keep getting crops of them until the attack has burnt itself out. It is worth persevering with treatment until they are all removed and it is important to ensure that your partner is treated at the same time to prevent re-infection.

Prevention of Sexually Transmitted Disease

1. You are more likely to contract STD when you have sex with a new partner. You don't, after all, know where he's been. It is wise, therefore, to use a sheath (or rather ask him to use one) during the early days of the relationship. Sheaths don't offer total protection but they do offer some and are much better than nothing.
2. If you do get an infection ensure that your partner is treated at the same time as you are.
3. Make sure that you complete a full course of treatment or infection may flare up again and be much more difficult to treat.

4. Forget the mythical toilet seats. All the infections dealt with in this chapter are sexually transmitted. The only infection you might possibly get from damp objects is trichomoniasis (see Chapter 6).

5. Keep both yourself and your vagina clean and healthy so that infections have less chance to take root. Wash carefully with clean water before you have sex and persuade your partner to do the same.

6. Venereologists dream of finding a vaccination to provide immunity against STD but it's a long way from being realised. Unlike other diseases, an attack of STD does not give you immunity. You can catch them again. So until the scientists in white coats solve the problem, it's really up to us to take extra care of ourselves and seek treatment immediately we suspect trouble.

Chapter Eight

Scabies and Pubic Lice

Lice, mites and other human parasites are as much a feature of life today as they have ever been. They are more controlled and less obvious than they were in the past but they still breed, feed and generally thrive on our bodies. Nor do they confine themselves to areas of social squalor but are quite happy to settle down on any human flesh available, irrespective of its background and social standing. So it is as well to know about them.

Crabs and Pubic Lice

Of all the creatures which feed on us, lice are the most unlovely and unloved. They are parasites which live exclusively on blood. So they can only survive if they are in close contact with the body and they are well adapted to escape capture. To pop a louse, you need a force 500,000 times its own weight.

There are two kinds of lice which live on humans and which are adapted to different areas of the body. One kind includes both the head louse and the body louse and the other is called *Pthirus pubis*, otherwise known as pubic lice or crabs.

Public lice are almost always transferred during sexual intercourse though they can occasionally be picked up from the bedding, clothes or towel of an infested person. They are called crabs because they look remarkably like crabs. They like coarse, wiry hair which is why they prefer to live in pubic hair. However, they can also be found under the arms, in beards and on eyelashes. They are very rarely found on children before puberty, for obvious reasons.

They are very small and extremely well camouflaged, but they can be seen with the naked eye and look like blueish-grey dots about the size of a pin head. They attach themselves to the roots of the pubic hair and insert their mouth parts into the skin to suck blood. This eventually causes intense itching which is the main symptom of infestation.

The females lay eggs or nits at a rate of five a day and these are cemented to the hair and hatch in a week. Since they can easily be transferred from one person to another, it is important to treat them quickly. This is a simple process and consists of using a cream, shampoo or powder such as Quellada which can be bought over the counter in the chemists or obtained free from a Special Clinic. Fortunately crabs do not like scalp hair but it is worth checking all your body hair if you are infested.

Use clean clothes and bedding after treatment. Crabs die within 24 hours if they don't feed but the nits can live for six days so it's necessary to see that all used clothing is either boiled, dry-cleaned or not used for a week.

Scabies

Scabies is caused by a mite known as *Sarcoptes scabiei* which is very contagious. Research conducted during the last world war showed that the mite is rarely caught from bedding and clothes but is passed on by prolonged intimate contact such as sleeping with an infected person. The researchers who discovered this fact composed the following piece of doggerel which Michael Andrews quotes in his book *The Life That Lives On Man*:

Recondite research on Sarcoptes
Has revealed that infections begin
On leave with your wives or your children
Or when you are living in sin.
Except in the case of the clergy
Who accomplish remarkable feats
And catch scabies and crabs
From door handles and cabs
And from blankets and lavatory seats

Scabies has been called 'the itch' because that is its chief symptom. There is a very, very itchy rash which is worse at night or when you are warm because that is when the mites become most active. Over 60 per cent of the mites burrow into the skin of the wrists or between the fingers but they can also be found on elbows, feet, ankles, buttocks and breasts.

The female mite burrows into the skin and lays eggs in the burrows which eventually hatch out and then make their way to the surface. In time these in turn burrow into the skin and lay their eggs and so on. The mite is not very nimble and moves slowly which is why it requires prolonged physical contact for them to transfer from one body to another. Once you have caught one, it will take four to six weeks before you feel any itching.

Treatment

The most effective treatment is to paint the skin with a benzyl benzoate solution which will be given to you at the clinic. This should be painted all over the body, especially in the skin folds. After two applications you will be told to have a hot bath and scrub the skin vigorously with soap and water. All clothes and towels should be washed and all members of the household should be checked to make sure that you are not infecting each other.

Chapter Nine

At the Neck of the Womb

The cervix is small, pink and rubbery. It connects the uterus to the vagina. Cervicitis is inflammation of the cervix. It is normally caused by some infection such as gonorrhoea, trichomonas, thrush or herpes. It usually causes a discharge and tenderness of the cervix which is probably most noticeable during intercourse. It can even cause back pains and abdominal pains. Sometimes an IUD string can cause inflammation, as can the chemicals in vaginal deodorants.

Cervicitis can be diagnosed either by taking a smear or from an internal examination which will show the cervix to be tender and swollen. Treatment will depend on what is causing the inflammation. Sometimes the problem is caused by a cervical erosion which has become infected.

Cervical Erosion

One of the worst things about a cervical erosion is its name. It sounds as though everything's breaking down and slipping away but that isn't what it means at all. What happens is that the cells from the inside canal of the cervix move onto the outside. An erosion looks like a small, reddish area near the entrance to the cervical canal.

Erosions are fairly common, especially in women who are on the Pill. They are not usually troublesome unless they start to produce a discharge or become infected. Occasionally there may be slight bleeding after intercourse.

If an erosion is not causing any symptoms it's probably wisest to leave it. If you stop taking the Pill it will usually go away. If you want to stay on the Pill and the erosion is causing a troublesome discharge or is responsible for recurrent infections, it can be cauterised or, more often, frozen off. This can be done in the out-patients' department of a hospital or even at a local clinic. It is not painful because there are very few nerve endings in the cervix:

> I was told as a result of a smear that I'd got a cervical erosion and inflammation, would I care to go back and see the doctor. I panicked and rushed back. She said it was very common, nothing to do with sexual activities, it occurs in nuns from time to time. She got rid of it the first time in order to take another smear. It was a fairly painless procedure. They just pop a little needle thing in, I hardly felt it, just a slight burning sensation but not enough to get upset about.

Polyps

Polyps are another condition which sounds much worse than it is. They are simply excessive growths of normal tissue which hang down, usually from the nose, cervix or womb. Cervical polyps are normally quite small and are not really painful. They may bleed after intercourse or during a routine examination. If they are troublesome, they can be removed fairly easily. Polyps which grow in the womb may prove more of a problem (see Chapter 10).

Cervical cancer

Cancer is a dreaded disease and not one most of us care to think about very much. Cervical cancer, however, is one form of the disease which can be treated successfully if it is detected early enough. This is why routine cervical smears are so important.

The tragedy is that not enough women, especially young women, have smears. The present NHS policy is that routine smears should be given every five years to women who are over 35 or who have had three or more pregnancies. Most doctors feel this is inadequate. In the last ten years, the number of deaths in the 25–34 age group has increased.

If you go to a Family Planning Clinic you will usually have a test as a matter of routine. You will also be tested when you are pregnant or at your post-natal examination. Otherwise you will have to ask your GP to test you or go to a

Well-Women clinic or a cytology (smear) clinic. *Women's National Cancer control Campaign* also runs mobile screening units which visit shopping areas and some large factories.

A smear test is the way in which doctors check for abnormal cells on the cervix. The body is made up of billions of tiny cells which are dying and being created all the time. Cancer occurs when the new cells grow abnormally and multiply too fast. In many parts of the body it is impossible to check what the cells are doing but fortunately the cervix is accessible.

It is not known exactly what causes cervical cancer but it has been established that it is connected to having sex with men. Nuns do not appear to suffer from the disease and it hasn't yet been recorded in a virgin. It is, however, common in prostitutes. It is also known that you have a much greater risk of developing cervical cancer if you start having sex under the age of eighteen, if you have babies very young and if you are promiscuous. For some reason middle-class women are less likely to develop it than working-class women and there is a possible connection with genital herpes (see Chapter 7). One theory behind all this is that some men carry a virus in their semen which affects the tissues of the cervix.

But whatever the reason, routine smears are the best protection for every woman. They are painless, free, and take less than ten minutes to do. You should go for a smear when you don't have a period and you should try not to use contraceptive foams or jellies for five days before you go, since these can alter the results.

The doctor will insert a cold metal speculum into your vagina and open it up to look at your cervix. S/he will then scrape a few loose cells from the cervix with a small, flat piece of wood. This smear is then sent to the laboratory where it is checked for abnormal cells.

The results of your test should be available in about two weeks. If all is well, you will have a negative result. If you have a positive result you will be asked to go back for another smear. This does not *necessarily* mean that you've got cancer so try not to panic if it happens. Any results at all which give rise to the slightest suspicion are sent back for a further check. Results which show the presence of infection such as trichomoniasis are also referred back to your doctor.

If your results show a mild abnormality you may just be asked to go back for another smear in a few months.

Mildly abnormal cells may never develop into cancer and can often go away by themselves. The important thing is to have frequent checks in case the abnormality develops into something which needs treating.

If you are found to have definitely pre-cancerous cells, you will be referred to a gynaecologist. S/he will give you a more thorough examination to check the cervix for abnormal cells. S/he will then decide what kind of treatment is necessary.

You may have a *punch biopsy* which means a tiny piece of the cervix is removed to be examined more thoroughly. This is usually done without anaesthetic, may hurt a little and bleed slightly afterwards. It is not, strictly speaking, a treatment, more an aid to accurate diagnosis.

Treatment usually takes the form of either destroying the affected area or removing it. In younger women doctors usually prefer to try and destroy the cancerous area. This is done either with heat treatment (*diathermy*) under general anaesthetic or with a cold treatment (*cryocautery*) which can be done in an out-patients' clinic. If you attend a very well equipped hospital, you may be treated by the new laser system.

Alternatively, if cancerous tissues are found, you will probably have a *cone biopsy*. This involves cutting a cone-shaped piece from the cervix, usually around the os where abnormal cells frequently begin. It is done under a general anaesthetic, but is not a painful operation to recover from.

A cone biopsy doesn't affect your ability to become pregnant but it does damage the cervix, making it very stiff and less able to dilate naturally. So if you become pregnant after you have had this operation you may need to be delivered by Caesarian section.

If you have *carcinoma in situ* (cancer which has not yet invaded the underlying tissues of the cervix) then the biopsy should remove all the abnormal cells though it is not always easy to tell. You will need to have regular smear tests afterwards to ensure all is well. In some cases the cancer may change and become *invasive*, i.e. it may start to invade other cells and grow inwards.

If the cancer is invasive, you will probably be advised to have a hysterectomy. This means the total surgical removal of the womb and it is a big operation with unpleasant side-effects. Sometimes doctors recommend a hysterectomy for any form of cervical cancer 'just in case' it becomes invasive. It is important that you find out from your doctor how advanced your cancer is before you consent to a hysterectomy, especially if you want more children.

The decision whether to risk your condition becoming invasive (which happens in about 20 per cent of cases) or whether to agree to a hysterectomy is an unenviable one but one which only you can make. Be sure that you understand exactly what is involved either way.

If the cancer is invasive when it is detected, you will almost certainly be advised to have a hysterectomy. This is a successful way of removing the cancer. If this is recommended, you will probably be given radiotherapy (X-ray treatment) as well. Radiotherapy has nasty side-effects like diarrhoea, vomiting and general weakness but is effective in killing cancer cells. Some women have found that taking Bio-Strath before, during and after a course of radiotherapy helps reduce the side-effects. Taking beetroot juice is also recommended because it helps keep your red blood corpuscle level high.

Each case of cervical cancer is highly individual, so you need to discuss the detail of your condition carefully with your doctor. Above all, it must be remembered that if the disease is detected in its early stages there is an almost 100 per cent certainty of cure. So look after yourself properly. A smear test today could save you much pain and anxiety tomorrow.

Chapter Ten

Womb Troubles

Womb means rather more than uterus though the two words refer to the same organ. The uterus is simply a bag of muscle which performs certain essential reproductive tasks. The womb is that which nurtures and nourishes, our first home and haven, a dark, hidden female centre. The trouble is that doctors tend to think in terms of the uterus and women in terms of the womb. This often causes considerable problems of communication, especially when it comes to the question of hysterectomy.

Hysterectomy

There is a great deal of confusion over exactly what is meant by a hysterectomy. Correctly it means the surgical removal of the whole uterus including the cervix but it is not used correctly very often. It may mean the removal of the main body of the uterus with the cervix being left. It may mean the removal of the uterus-plus-cervix-plus ovaries and tubes. It is therefore *very* important if your doctor recommends a hysterectomy that you find out exactly what s/he believes should be removed and why.

There are too many hysterectomies performed in this country. Some doctors believe that when a woman has completed her family, she has no more use for her uterus and therefore it might as well be removed. Women, however, often regard their womb as an important part of their sexuality. If you feel that way, then tell your doctor how you feel and ask if there is any alternative treatment for your condition. There may not be, but at least you will be sure that your womb is not being removed just to make life simpler for the doctor. If you have a doctor who isn't prepared to discuss the matter with you, remember that you are entitled to get a second opinion.

Hysterectomies should never be used as an abortion method. Nor should you accept one as a method of sterilisation; sealing off the tubes is a much safer operation. If you have fibroids much will depend on how large and extensive they are (see Fibroids). Insist that your ovaries remain unless you are given an excellent reason for their removal. Your ovaries secrete small amounts of oestrogen which help you through the menopause. If they are removed the after-effects of the surgery can be much more difficult.

A hysterectomy is a major operation with all the attendant risks from shock and anaesthetics. You will probably suffer from quite severe pain after the operation and it will take three or four months to recover.

How you react to the surgery emotionally will depend very much on what is wrong with you and what your symptoms were before the operation. It has been found that women who suffer the operation for fairly minor reasons become much more depressed afterwards than women who suffer it because there is something serious wrong. Much will depend, also, on how important your womb is to your sense of being female. Certainly depression is one of the most common complications of the operation. So it really is vital that you discuss how you feel about the operation with close friends and family before you make a decision about having it done.

Fibroids

Around 20 to 25 per cent of women over the age of thirty have fibroids. They are benign (not dangerous) growths composed of muscle and fibrous tissue. They usually grow in clusters but they grow very slowly and more often than not women don't know they have any.

It is thought that fibroids grow in response to stimulation from oestrogen but nobody knows for sure. Sometimes the Pill may cause them to grow more quickly, but this is not always the case. Once oestrogen levels drop after the menopause, fibroids will cease to grow and may even shrink.

Occasionally fibroids may block the Fallopian tubes and cause infertility. During pregnancy they tend to grow more quickly because of the increased oestrogen levels. If they bulge into the cavity of the uterus they may leave the baby too little room to grow and precipitate a miscarriage. Or if they block the birth canal they may make delivery difficult. However, they are usually too small to cause such problems. After childbirth the fibroids shrink back to the size they were before pregnancy.

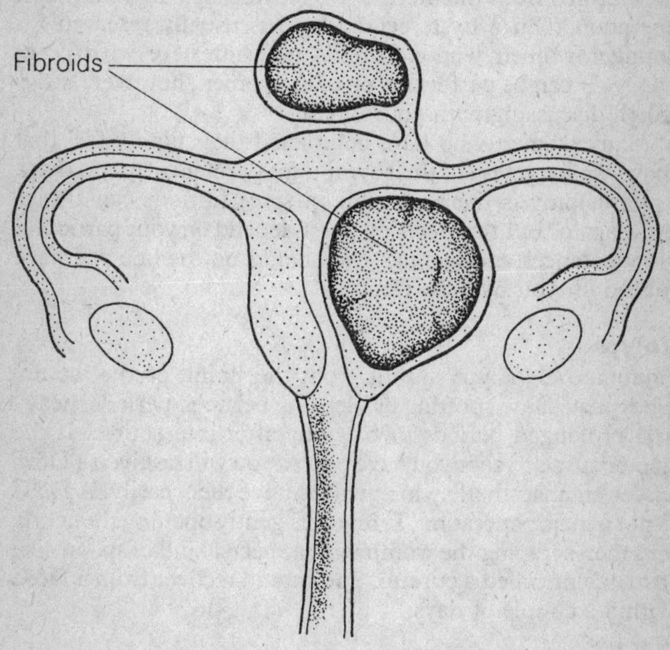

Fibroids only cause serious problems when they become large enough to interfere with other bodily functions. If they bulge into the cavity of the uterus, you may find you develop heavy periods which last much longer than usual. If they press against the bladder wall or rectal wall they may cause problems with emptying your bladder properly (which can lead to infection) or upset normal bowel movements. They don't normally cause pain though they may create a feeling of heaviness in the pelvic area and occasionally backache.

Treatment

If your fibroids are small and not causing you any trouble, then it's much better to leave them well alone. If they are large and causing trouble you may wish to consider surgery.

It is possible to have surgery which leaves the uterus in place. This is called a *myomectomy* and involves the removal of the fibroids from the uterus. It is technically a more difficult operation than a hysterectomy and is usually reserved for younger women whose fibroids may interfere with pregnancy. It can be performed on older women, however, and is worth discussing with your doctor.

Many women who have completed their family feel that they want to get rid of their symptoms permanently and that a hysterectomy is the best solution since fibroids can always grow again. But this decision must depend on your particular circumstances and feelings and should not be one you have foisted on you by a doctor.

Polyps

Endometrial polyps sprout from the lining of the womb. They may cause spotting or bleeding between periods, heavy and prolonged periods or bleeding after intercourse. If the doctor suspects that you have polyps you will be given a D&C under an anaesthetic which will remove them easily. A D&C is not a major operation. It involves gently opening the cervix and then scraping the womb with a special kind of spoon-like instrument called a curette. You should recover from a D&C within a couple of days.

Prolapse

A prolapse occurs when the muscles which support the uterus begin to sag. As a result the uterus slowly descends into the vaginal canal. This may lead to a heavy, dragging sensation in the lower abdomen or low backache.

Prolapse of the uterus used to be a much more common problem when women were worn out by constant pregnancies. It can still happen today but you will help yourself avoid it if you exercise your pelvic floor muscles. This is especially important after childbirth when the muscles are stretched and slack but it should be continued regularly thereafter to keep the muscles good and firm.

The exercises are easy to do and can be performed any time, anywhere without attracting attention. Those endless queues at bus stops, post-office counters and the checkout at the supermarket are ideal places to practise.

To discover your pelvic floor muscles try and stop the flow of urine when you are next on the loo. If you can completely stop it then your muscles are well tensed. Then relax and the urine will flow again. Once you are aware of the muscles and how to control them you can practise the exercises every day. This should be done by contracting the muscles tight, holding the contraction for three seconds and then relaxing slowly.

Ideally you should do two hundred or so contractions each day to keep the muscles in tip-top shape but you don't really need to count, just practise regularly. You will find that if you do, one of the added advantages is that it adds an extra pzaz to lovemaking since the ability to make your vagina nice and tight during intercourse improves sensation for both partners. And since most of us worry about developing a slack vagina, these exercises can relieve much anxiety.

If you do develop a prolapse, however, you don't need to suffer in silence. Surgery can correct the problem by repairing the sagging supports for your uterus. Or you may be offered a hysterectomy which you may, or may not, feel is necessary. Again, the decision is yours though it is helpful if you can discuss all the alternatives thoroughly with your doctor.

Endometrial Cancer

Cancer of the lining of the uterus is, fortunately, quite rare. Women who are most at risk are usually over fifty, have a history of irregular periods and have probably found it difficult to become pregnant. It has also been found that being overweight, having high blood pressure and diabetes are common factors in women who develop this form of cancer. This has led some experts to believe the condition may be inherited. Hormone replacement therapy is also under suspicion as a cause (see Chapter 3). It seems that in some women the uterine lining is hypersensitive to the effects of oestrogen.

Since this form of cancer usually develops in older women, the most common symptom is spotting or bleeding after the menopause. The bleeding need not be heavy. But any woman who has not had a period for over a year and who develops any bleeding, however slight, should have it investigated as soon as possible. If cancer of the uterus is diagnosed early it is almost 100 per cent curable.

In younger women who are still menstruating the symptoms will include grossly irregular periods and/or bleeding or spotting between periods. These are symptoms for a number of conditions but you should always have them investigated.

The only way to effectively diagnose cancer of the uterus is for the doctor to perform a D&C and then examine the cells which have been removed. If you do have cancer you will almost certainly need a hysterectomy including the removal of your tubes and ovaries. It is necessary to remove the ovaries because they may have hidden tumours. They also produce oestrogen which can stimulate cancer cells. Alternative treatments include radiation therapy and hormone treatment with a progesterone-like hormone.

Endometriosis

Endometriosis is a condition which happens when parts of the lining of the uterus (endometrium) leak and spread outside the uterus. Usually it spreads up the Fallopian tubes and onto the ovaries. Because this endometrial tissue is hormone-sensitive it will continue to behave as it did in the uterus. In other words it will swell, thicken and bleed and then shrink until the next cycle. If the blood which is shed has nowhere to go it forms scabs or clots and scar tissue which can distend the tubes and cause pain or cause a cyst on the ovary.

Endometriosis is not very common. It is estimated that between 5 to 10 per cent of women suffer from it. These are usually women between the ages of 25 and 45. But it is very unpleasant if you do have it. Its main symptoms are increasingly painful periods, usually experienced as a dull, nagging pain in the lower abdomen, and severe pain during sexual intercourse. It also causes infertility in a number of cases by binding up the Fallopian tubes and preventing them from working.

Your doctor may suspect you have the condition from the symptoms you suffer and a pelvic examination. But it might be necessary for you to have a *laparoscopy*. This is done either with a general or a local anaesthetic and involves a visual inspection of your pelvic organs. A needle is inserted under the skin and into the deeper parts of the abdomen. Carbon dioxide is then blown through the needle which puffs out the abdomen. A tiny telescope-like instrument is then inserted and the ovaries, tubes and uterus are examined. Sometimes a dye is injected into the uterus through the cervix. If this dye reaches the end of the Fallopian tubes it proves that they are clear, otherwise they are seen to be blocked. When the investigation is over the gas is allowed to escape through a tiny cut which is made near the navel. The operation may be slightly uncomfortable but you will recover within a week or so. This is a much more effective method of diagnosis than any other:

> Anyway, he said that he wanted me in for this laparoscopy. They stick the needle in and look down at the ovaries. I went into hospital and had this done. They confirmed that I had endometriosis. The problem was that with me, instead of the blood actually forming into pockets where they could have operated and scraped it away, it had soaked into the muscular wall of the womb. So there was nothing they could do about it.
>
> He put me on a course of hormones. They stop you having periods altogether, but it wasn't like the pill. He said it was the male hormone. It was incredibly expensive. Each tablet cost two pounds and I was taking two a day. I took these things for three months. I put weight on and I lost about two inches off my bust. I didn't grow a beard, luckily. Anyway, after three months he said I could come off the pills and my weight began to drop. And, so far, I haven't had any further trouble.

The chief method of treatment is some form of hormone therapy which will stop both periods and ovulation. In many cases this is very effective. Some women, however, suffer very unpleasant side-effects and in other cases the condition recurs once the hormone pills are stopped.

Minor surgery is also possible, especially if your tubes are affected and you wish to have children. This surgery involves the scraping away and removal of the leaked endometrial tissue. If you do have surgery it should be accompanied by hormone therapy to prevent the condition recurring. If you become pregnant, of course, the effect is the same as hormone therapy and often pregnancy can clear up the condition completely.

In a small number of women, however, the pain persists and interferes with their lives. If that is the case, it may be necessary for you to have radical surgery in order to get permanent relief. This would involve the removal of the uterus and sometimes even the ovaries. Fortunately this is rarely necessary, especially if the condition is diagnosed in its early stages.

Chapter Eleven

Tubes and Ovaries

Salpingitis

I must confess that I had not intended to do any first-hand research when I started writing this book. Nonetheless, I found myself a few months ago, laid up with salipingitis. And I can report that it is indeed a very unpleasant experience.

Salpingitis is an inflammation of the Fallopian tubes. It is one of the conditions which often passes under the umbrella term 'pelvic inflammatory disease' (PID). When doctors use the term PID, what they usually mean is that they know that some part of the pelvic organs is inflamed but can't easily tell which part. The following information on salpingitis, therefore, is equally valid for PID if that's the label you're given for your pain.

The condition can have varying degrees of severity. In my case, since it occurred just after Christmas, I put it down to all kinds of over-indulgence. The pain was dull and low down. I rested in the belief that it would sort itself out which it didn't. Four days later the pain was so bad I was convinced it was appendicitis. In fact, the sharp pain of salpingitis in its acute form is often mistaken for appendicitis even by doctors. So if you have it this badly you will find it impossible to get out of bed and you will probably be running a fever of about 100^0 – 102^0F. You may also have vomiting and nausea.

An attack need not be this severe, however. It can occur as a few mild bouts of abdominal pain or cramps over a period of several weeks or months. The pain may coincide with the beginning of a period, or in some cases, at the time of ovulation. You may also find that you have pain during sexual intercourse, irregular periods or low backache. The pain usually eases if you rest but is really bad if you do anything physically strenuous. If the infection is caused by gonorrhoea there may be a vaginal discharge and you will probably have a slight fever of about 90°F. If you don't seek treatment at this stage, things can only get worse.

The most dangerous and worrying thing about salpingitis is that if the infection is not cleared up quickly it can block or seal the tubes with scar tissue. This may lead either to infertility or to ectopic pregnancy.

Causes

All kinds of bacteria can cause an inflammation of the tubes. The most common are E-coli (of cystitis fame), streptococci and gonococci (as in gonorrhoea). Infection usually travels upwards from the vagina, cervix or uterus. You are most vulnerable to infection if your body resistance is low or if your uterus is made vulnerable as a result of childbirth, abortion or IUD insertion. IUD strings are, in fact, a positive magnet for all kinds of infection. The chief danger, however, occurs when you have one inserted because the uterus is then exposed to any infection around. It has been estimated that IUD users have about five times the risk of catching pelvic infections as non-users.

If you have only a mild attack of salpingitis it can easily be wrongly diagnosed, especially if your doctor doesn't examine you. If you have any suspicion at all either ask your doctor to do an examination or go to a clinic and have one. It really isn't wise to hang around and await developments with this condition. If you suspect that you might have gonorrhoea it is important to tell the doctor so that s/he can do the proper tests. Occasionally you may be given a laparoscopy (see Chapter 10) if there is some doubt as to the diagnosis.

Treatment

Treatment is usually with antibiotics but it is *vital* that you rest. One week in bed at the very least is essential. Eat well and avoid sex until the infection has cleared. If you have been given the correct antibiotics your symptoms should clear within a few days. If they don't then see your doctor again and try a different antibiotic.

Some women find that a hot water bottle laid on the sore

area is blissfully soothing. Relaxation is certainly essential or you will tense up, make the pain worse and stop the blood flowing properly to the infected area. So home help is vital or, failing that, a short stay in hospital may be the answer if your attack is acute.

Unfortunately, some women find that antibiotics are not very effective and the infection flares up again once they have finished the first course. If this happens and you suffer from recurrent bouts of pelvic infection it is probably a good idea to have a proper investigation done so that the doctor can tell exactly what bacteria is causing the infection.

If you have suffered an attack of salpingitis, you should avoid using an IUD and use the Pill if possible. If for some reason you can't take the Pill, then use a cap or sheath and some form of spermicide. This is necessary because there is a danger of ectopic pregnancy if your tubes have been scarred and an ectopic pregnancy can be very dangerous. The coil does not prevent the fertilisation of an egg, it simply prevents it from implanting in the wall of the uterus, so you need to use a contraceptive method which prevents fertilisation.

Ectopic pregnancy

Ectopic is a medical word meaning outside its proper site. An ectopic pregnancy is one which occurs outside the uterus. What happens is that the egg is fertilised in the Fallopian tube but if the tube is narrowed or twisted by some infection, the fertilised egg is unable to travel down to the uterus. It therefore begins to grow and develop into the damaged tube. As the embryo enlarges it stretches the tube and eventually the tube bursts. This causes severe internal bleeding and if you do not receive immediate medical care your life is at risk.

The first symptoms of an ectopic pregnancy are the same as for a normal pregnancy. In the early stages it is very difficult to detect that the embryo is growing in the wrong place. Within two weeks of the missed period, you may find some light spotting or bleeding. The tube is likely to burst between the 10th and 14th week. Just before it does you may feel a stabbing pain or cramps or a constant dull abdominal pain because the tube is so stretched.

Once you start to bleed inside the pain will increase in the lower abdomen and you are likely to develop the most distinctive feature of all, which is shoulder-tip pain. It's thought this is caused by blood flowing up to your diaphragm. You may find your breathing is painful and if there is a great deal of blood-loss you will probably have symptoms of shock with low blood pressure, a high pulse rate, hot and cold flushes, nausea, dizziness or fainting. At this point you are in need of emergency attention. As one doctor explained to me:

> You usually find it when you've got a patient coming into Casualty flat on her back, having collapsed with not a lot of blood lost vaginally and much more shocked and distressed than she out to be. Then she says, 'I feel dreadful, I've got tummy ache and I don't know why my shoulder hurts.' That's when the casualty officer will prick his ears up.
>
> She may collapse very unexpectedly. She thinks she's pregnant, may even have had the pregnancy confirmed. Then she may get a little vaginal bleeding and may have already gone to bed thinking it's a threatened miscarriage. She then suddenly starts to feel very unwell with a severe stomach ache or one-sided pain and then she collapses and is very shocked and probably in quite a lot of pain.

Once you arrive in hospital with an ectopic pregnancy you will receive immediate surgery to remove the burst tube and transfusions to replace the lost blood. After you have had one tube removed, you halve your chances of conceiving again, but if your other tube is healthy you will still be able to have a baby.

Ectopic pregnancies can occur, however, in women who have no history of pelvic infections so all pregnant women should be aware of the symptoms and see their doctor if they have any cause for suspicion. If you have suffered from salpingitis this is especially important as you will be more at risk.

Ovarian cysts

There are ovarian cysts and ovarian cysts. The most common

type are usually small, come and go of their own accord and don't give much trouble. There are other types, however, which grow to the size of a grapefruit or even a football and they, obviously, need to be surgically removed.

A cyst develops when a follicle has ripened, as they do each month in preparation for ovulation, but has failed to burst and release an egg. Most cysts fill with fluid but some are solid. They can grow very quickly and if they do the symptoms they are likely to produce are an unexplained swelling of the abdomen, pain during intercourse or disrupted periods. Sometimes women also develop a pain in their leg as this woman did:

> The really weird thing is that I had a pain in my leg on and off for two years. I told the doctor about it and he said, 'Oh, it's nerves or something.' Everything was nervous. But later I talked to a friend who had exactly the same thing.'

In fact pelvic pain is often felt in the legs. This can happen with period pains and there are women who experience labour pain entirely in their thighs.

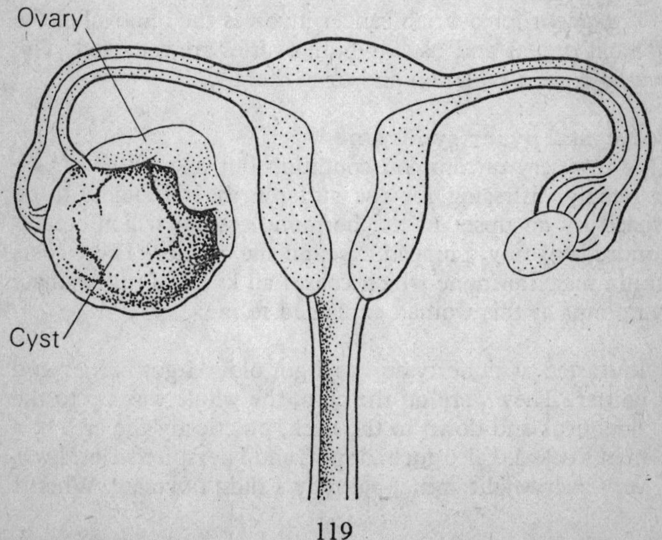

If you have a large ovarian cyst it will probably be benign but it may be dangerous and in either case it will probably need to be removed. The only way for the doctor to judge properly is to perform a laparoscopy. If the cyst is benign it can be removed leaving the remaining part of the ovary still working.

Cancer of the Ovaries

Ovarian cancer is much rarer than cancer of the cervix or uterus but it is also more dangerous. It tends to occur most frequently in women past the menopause but can occur in younger women. The problem with this form of cancer is that once malignant tumours develop they spread very rapidly. And since there are no early symptoms women have no way of knowing this is happening.

There is no really effective way of screening for ovarian cancer. The first symptoms are likely to be the swelling and abdominal pain which occur with any ovarian cysts. Only investigation can show whether a growth on the ovary is malignant or not. If you are past the menopause it is worth having a pelvic examination at regular invervals when any lumps on the ovaries can be detected and investigated.

Treatment for ovarian cancer involves the removal of the affected organs and usually both ovaries are removed. You may also need radiation and drug therapy.

Polycystic ovary syndrome

This is a very uncommon condition but one which can be extremely distrssing for the sufferer. It is thought to be caused by an upset in the hormone system which creates hundreds of tiny, pinhead cysts on the ovaries. These cysts emit a male hormone which causes all kinds of unfortunate symptoms as this woman explained to me:

> It started at puberty and as I got older I got hairier and hairier. They were on the chin, the whole way up to the sideburns and down to the neck, practically the area of a man's beard. I also got bad spots and I perspired a lot. I was very overweight and apparently I didn't ovulate. When I

first went to the doctor he said, 'Don't be silly dear, you'll grow out of it,' but I didn't. Luckily I was later referred to the endocrinology department at Barts Hospital where it was treated.

Treatment for this condition is usually hormone pills plus electrolysis to deal with the facial hair. It is always worth remembering that these strange hormonal disorders do occur. Persist with your quest for treatment if you are initially fobbed off by your GP.

Chapter Twelve

After Birth

Having a baby is a major unheaval in any woman's life, to put it mildly. The upheaval is both emotional and physical and the two usually interact. The result, all too often, is a feeling of soreness, exhaustion, weepiness, loss of confidence or downright depression. Depression is the most common complication of the period following childbirth. Its causes are too complex to cover here. My earlier book on the subject deals with them in detail. There are, however, certain purely physical problems which add to the load of stress women have to carry at this time. These can and should be reduced to a minimum.

Episiotomy

An episiotomy is a cut in the perineum which is made at the time of delivery. It has been called 'the unkindest cut' because the perineum is such an incredibly sensitive sexual area. Indeed, many women describe their episiotomy as much the worst part of the whole birth experience.

Doctors claim that episiotomies are necessary to prevent tearing. A cut is cleaner and easier to stitch than a jagged, untidy tear. Unfortunately, however, they are increasingly performed in most hospitals as a matter of routine rather than clinical judgement. There are very few women who escape one.

In fact, if the baby's head is allowed a slow delivery and the perineum is carefully massaged, there is no reason why it should tear. In Holland where almost half of all births occur at home with a midwife in attendance, the number of episiotomies performed is minute compared to this country.

Doctors tend to treat episiotomy as a small, rather insignificant operation but it is far from that for the woman concerned. Pain in this area makes it impossible to be really comfortable whether standing, sitting or lying. Sometimes the pain can be so bad that we lose interest in our babies, blaming them as being the cause of the pain. Almost certainly we lose interest in sex since even the thought of it brings twinges of agony.

All this is bad enough if the cut has been stitched properly. Unfortunately this isn't always the case. Often stitching is left to an inexperienced medical student who may make a botched job of it. As one GP explained to me:

> Sometimes you see a piece of stitching that was done by a student on his first try and it's terrible. I mean fundamental things like the layers of the tissues have been stuck together wrong. It can be terribly painful. So you sent the woman back for an appointment and tell them to start again. That's the only thing you can do isn't it? Undo all the bad work and re-stitch it.

There is no point in worrying whether you've been ruined for life by bad stitching. You have to ask a doctor to check the stitches for you after they've been done if you're suspicious. And if they go on feeling very painful you must go on asking for reassurance.

To ease the pain of the stitches, there is nothing to beat a salt bath. If you are in hospital it isn't always easy to have as many of these as you'd like, but once you get home you should really indulge yourself. Salt doesn't sting the wound when it is mixed with water, on the contrary, it is amazingly soothing. If you don't have time for a lot of baths you can always sit in a bowl or baby bath full of salt water. You may also find that sitting on a rubber ring helps ease the pain of stitches because it takes the weight off the sore spot.

You don't need to rush into lovemaking again at the earliest opportunity, but nor do you need to avoid it. Many women need to feel that they are still attractive and desirable as females after they have had babies. Play the whole thing by touch as far as possible and talk to your partner about how you feel. He may expect you to bounce back to normal straight away or he may feel very anxious and concerned not to hurt you. You won't know unless you ask him.

If you find that you are very sore, then remember that it is possible to make love without having intercourse, oral or manual stimulation can be as loving and as satisfying. And when you do feel able to resume intercourse again, remember that your vagina is likely to be rather dry, so you will need plenty of KY jelly. It is also sensible to experiment with positions so that the scar tissue isn't rubbed too much whilst it is still tender. If you have any anxieties about the shape and texture of your vagina, then examine it yourself and if you still feel unhappy go and see your GP or go to a clinic and be checked.

Exhaustion

If you haven't been heavily drugged, you will probably find that immediately after birth you feel incredibly excited. This may last for a couple of days and then you are likely to have a reaction, feeling really tired and possibly weepy. When this happens you need to find someone you can talk to who will support you. You also need to sleep as much as possible.

If you are in hospital you may feel that the hospital routine prevents you from being able to relax and sleep when you want to. Popular wisdom has it that a stay in hospital gives you a chance to rest but many women find the opposite. If you can't rest in hospital and if you have friends or family prepared to come and help out with the housework, you can ask to be discharged as soon as possible. You may have to be very firm about it because hospitals seem to like hanging on to patients once they have them inside. If it comes to it, you can always discharge yourself.

Once you are back at home, the important thing to avoid is being entirely on your own coping with the new baby all day. If you have other children, it is even more important to have help. It takes time to come to terms emotionally with the fact of having a new member of the family and babies can be very demanding.

The golden rule is to expect yourself to be pretty useless at the job of motherhood for the first few months anyway. That way you won't fall into the terrible trap of trying to prove how perfect you are. Everyone finds this postnatal period exhausting and difficult and you need to use all the help you can get.

Your concentration and energy should be going into getting to know the baby and making sure that you recover and rest from the birth. Everything else is secondary. Explain to your partner that although giving birth is a natural process, it is an exhausting and stressful natural process, rather like running the Marathon. You need to be allowed to recover your strength if you are to be of any use to anyone. This means that he will have to help with the cleaning, washing, shopping and cooking for a few months and the practise will be good for him. If it is humanly possible, you should keep your activities to the minimum.

Night-feeding is not only tiring, it can also be very disorientating. It is easy to forget both the time of the day and the day of the week when you never get a night's uninterrupted sleep. If you are breast-feeding you may feel especially tied but in fact it doesn't do any harm for the baby to be given one bottle a day (or in the night) so that you can get that precious long sleep. Some women also find it easier to sleep either with the baby in bed with them, or in a basket next to the bed, so that they don't have to wake up fully to feed him or her.

If you have other children then they probably have friends who have mothers who know exactly how you feel. Don't be ashamed to ask these mothers to take your older children for an afternoon or even the week-end. When you are fit and bouncy again, you can return the favour. If you don't know anyone, or are trying to cope on your own, talk to your Health Visitor and see if she can arrange any kind of home help. It's all too easy to be proud, stick your chin in the air and say 'I can cope', but if you do that now, you may find that in a few months you're too depressed even to cope with getting out of bed.

After having a baby your body has to handle a number of very considerable changes before it can begin to function smoothly again. It needs all the help you can give it to help it re-adjust. If you don't eat properly or allow yourself to become exhausted you will undermine your body's resistance to infection and make its re-adjustment that much more difficult. You owe it to yourself to really look after yourself at this time.

Anaemia

Anaemia is due to a shortage of red-blood cells. This may happen either because you have lost a great deal of blood or because there is a drop in the haemoglobin level. Blood checks in pregnancy ensure that doctors know if you are developing anaemia but once you are at home with the baby no further checks are made so it is something which you need to watch for yourself.

If you find you have unusually heavy bleeding, heavier than a normal period on any day, then rest straight away and see a doctor as soon as you can. It is possible to have a secondary post-partum haemorrage anything up to six weeks after delivery if you are too active too soon. A heavy loss of blood should always be attended to.

Otherwise, the symptoms of anemia are very similar to those of the post-natal period generally. They include extreme tiredness, impatience, shortness of breath, lethargy and pallor, especially of the nails, lips and the inside of the lower eyelid.

The best way to prevent anaemia developing is to eat food which is rich in calcium, iron and vitamin C and B.

If this proves too difficult to organise, then you should take iron and vitamin tablets for at least three months after delivery. The only accurate way of detecting anaemia is by having a blood test. So if you have a good reason to suspect you might be anaemic you should go and consult your doctor about it.

Other Physical Complications

Partial retained placenta

The placenta should always be very carefully checked after delivery to ensure that it has all come away. Occasionally, however, small pieces may be left in the uterus and this can cause quite serious problems. If this happens you may find that about two weeks (or sometimes even longer) after delivery you start bleeding quite heavily and may be passing blood clots. The discharge is likely to be a blackish-brown with a horrible smell. You may also have some abdominal pain:

> It was a few weeks after the baby was born. There were lumps coming away and it was smelling so I went to Casualty. They sent me back to the hospital where I had him. There I was examined and they said I had to come in straight away, that same day. They gave me a D & C and said that part of the afterbirth had been removed.

Since this is the commonest cause of uterine infection after birth it is important to have treatment immediately if you suspect anything. A piece of placenta left in the uterus provides an ideal breeding ground for bacteria.

Uterine infections

You are very vulnerable to infection after having a baby since bacteria find blood an ideal breeding ground and your uterus is more open and less protected than it would normally be. The symptoms are the same as those for any pelvic infection (see Chapter 10) with the addition that your lochia discharge is likely to be more profuse and smellier than before.

In the past uterine infection was the cause of puerperal fever and was a killer. Today it can be treated with antibiotics, but not easily, and you really are laid up with it. It's necessary to be very careful indeed about your personal hygeine. Have a salt bath at least once a day. Salt cleanses as well as soothes wounds. And change your pads regularly. Avoid any chemical irritants like the plague.

Urinary problems

If you have had a long and difficult labour, or a forceps delivery, you may develop cystitis after the baby has been born. The best way of handling this is by the self-help methods described in Chapter 5. You should consult a doctor in case there is an infection present. If your bladder has been bruised, you may find that you are incontinent for a time. This can make life difficult but the bladder recovers fairly quickly.

Chapter Thirteen

About Sex

Most of us grow up knowing very little about our sexuality. It's an area of our lives where we tend to learn by trial and error. There's no reason why we should, of course, since there are now plenty of books about sex on the market telling us everything we could possibly need to know. The main trouble is that when it actually comes down to it we are far more influenced by the attitudes towards sex which we meet as children than we are by the theory we read as adults.

Anxiety is a great passion killer. Many sexual problems occur either because we don't feel relaxed and happy about our bodies so we tense up or because we find it hard to talk about our sexual feelings which we think might be 'wrong'. Either way the problem only gets worse if it's ignored. It's so easy to get strange ideas about what sex 'ought' to be when really what matters is what you find satisfying.

To explore all the difficulties which can arise as a result of anxiety and emotional hang-ups would take a book in itself. There are, however, certain physical conditions which can affect our sexual satisfaction and these are worth examining.

Female sexual response

Women get turned on by different things at different times depending on our mood, how tired we feel, what time of the month it is and how effective the stimulus is. But once we do begin to feel aroused our physical response follows the same basic pattern.

Our first response to effective sexual stimulation is a moist vagina. Once we feel excited the vaginal walls secrete a lubricating fluid very rapidly and continue doing so as long as the excitement continues. As stimulation continues, more and more blood is pumped into the pelvic area. This leads to an engorgement of the tissues. In some women the womb can actually double in size during sexual arousal. The labia minora (inner lips) thicken, the clitoris swells and the upper part of the vagina closest to the cervix begins to widen and lengthen. The rest of the body also responds with an increased pulse rate, heavy breathing and nipple erection.

As tension mounts, the mouth of the vagina tightens, the clitoris draws back into its hood and the labia minora change colour from light pink to deep red. Orgasm occurs as a kind of seizure of tension-releasing rhythmic contractions of the womb and lower vagina. The stronger the orgasm, the more numerous are the contractions.

Following orgasm the body begins to return to normal. This happens much more quickly to men than to women and women are able to experience several orgasms within a short space of time. Orgasm permits all the blood which has filled the tissues of the pelvic area to drain away.

Pelvic congestion

If we are consistently aroused and fail to reach orgasm we will suffer from pelvic congestion because the blood takes hours to dissipate. Pelvic congestion leads to abdominal discomfort, backache, tension and irritability. It can also interfere with normal sleep. Obviously there are occasions when all of us fail to reach orgasm without suffering too much damage. It is the woman who rarely experiences orgasm after arousal who needs to tackle the problem in earnest.

There are so many strange ideas and feelings about female orgasm that it may take a long time to really sort out what the problem is. Many women believe that the normal pattern is for orgasm to occur at the same time for both partners. In fact this happens so rarely that it is the exception rather than the rule. If you wait for it to happen you are likely to be left stranded, blaming yourself for your lack of satisfaction and feeling very guilty and anxious.

Many women also worry about masturbation, feeling that it is something unnatural and wrong. This is an old belief which was created by the Victorian medical profession. The Kinsey report exposed it as a myth by proving that masturbation is the most universal and common form of human sexual activity.

Pelvic congestion will only be relieved by orgasm and how you set about achieving orgasm depends entirely on you and your partner. Every couple is different and it's a matter of trying to discover what gives both of you satisfaction. Women have sexual needs too and shouldn't feel guilty about working to satisfy them.

Painful intercourse

Pain during intercourse may be felt either at the mouth of the vagina or in the pelvis during deep penetration. There are a number of physical conditions which can be responsible for either kind of pain.

Pain at the entrance to the vagina is usually caused by either insufficient vaginal lubrication or inflammation due to a vaginal infection. If the vagina is not moist enough at the time of penetration, the friction of the penis can be very painful and can irritate the bladder causing cystitis to flare up. A water-soluble lubricating jelly such as KY jelly can help. Don't use vaseline, especially if you are using a condom or cap as a contraceptive, it rots rubber and isn't too good for flesh.

Sometimes dryness is caused by a lack of oestrogen. This happens especially after childbirth and after the menopause. Lack of oestrogen effects the vaginal walls in such a way that they produce less moisture during arousal. If this is a serious problem your doctor can give you vaginal suppositories or hormone therapy. Otherwise lubricating jelly should be sufficient to see you through.

The most common cause of vaginal dryness, however, is lack of stimulation. You simply aren't aroused enough when penetration occurs. This may be due to anxiety, an over-eager partner or simply lack of interest. If you find that you are rarely aroused, it is worth taking a good look at your life to see why it lacks excitement. If we get bogged down in housework and child-rearing routines it is easy to get over-tired and bored with life. Sexual excitement is psychological and can only occur if we enjoy being who we are and feel in touch with life. Which is why we owe it to ourselves to make time and space for our own interests and our own pleasure.

Tightness of the vaginal entrance may be due to an unstretched hymen in a young woman in which case the hymen can gently be stretched with a finger. If you use a mirror to look at your vulva you should be able to see where the hymen is and stretch it yourself. The vaginal opening also tenses up if you are anxious and not yet ready for penetration, so don't allow yourself to be rushed.

Stinging, irritation or burning feelings at the opening to the vagina are often caused by a vaginal infection such as thrush or trichomoniasis (see Chapter 6) Or your vagina may have been irritated by some chemical spray or deodorant or by the birth control cream, jelly or foam you are using.

Pain felt deep in the pelvis during penetration is almost always due to some form of medical condition. Endometriosis (see Chapter 10) is noted for causing a sharp, stabbing pain on penetration. Any infections of the cervix, tubes or uterus will cause pain as will the presence of cysts on the ovaries. All these conditions should receive medical attention. Sometimes it is painful when the penis hits the cervix. This can be prevented either by a change of position (the rear-engry position with your buttocks facing your partner can help) or by limiting the depth of penetration.

If you find that you have any pain during intercourse then you should go to your doctor for a check. If your doctor is unwilling to examine you then go to a Well-Woman clinic. It is important to check that your problems are not physical before you start worrying about your psychology. It is also worth remembering that gynaecologists are not trained to deal with sexual problems so any advice they may give you on the subject which isn't strictly physical is just their own opinion, may well be biased and should be taken with a pinch of salt.

Sex after a hysterectomy

A hysterectomy does not physically affect your ability to have sex. The vagina should not be shortened if the operation has been properly done. Despite this, some women do complain that their vagina is too short after the operation. If you feel this has happened you must go back to your doctor and have it checked. If your ovaries have been removed with your uterus you may find that you produce less vaginal lubrication which should be dealt with as indicated earlier in this chapter.

Vaginismus

Vaginismus is a physical condition caused by an emotional problem. What happens is that the muscles of the outer third of the vagina tighten in an involuntary spasm, making penetration impossible. This is a means whereby the body defends itself from a sexual situation which you find unconsciously threatening. Often it has to do with feelings of being powerless or controlled by other people. It may happen as the result of a traumatic experience such as rape but it can equally happen for no clearly obvious reason.

Women who suffer from vaginismus very often feel complete failures and may avoid any attempt at sex. It can be a dreadfully humiliating experience. Medical treatment for the problem varies. Gynaecological treatment which attempts to enlarge the vagina is not really much use. Behaviour therapy tackles the symptom by teaching women muscle relaxation and gently introducing dilators into the vagina. This is an attempt to help them to unlearn this particular response to anxiety. It can be helpful but there is always the risk that the anxiety will break out again with different symptoms. Good psychotherapy can be useful in tackling the causes of the anxiety but it can take a long time and it tends to be expensive. Talking to close friends and coming to terms with the fact that you have a problem which you really want to solve can often be a good way of beginning. Thereafter it's a matter of trying what therapy is offered and using what you find helpful.

One woman I talked to suffered from vaginisimus only when she was being examined by male doctors which presented her with a very difficult situation:

> It first happened when I was about eighteen and my own GP wanted to examine me after a miscarriage. He wasn't

particularly threatening, it was just that he made me feel that I didn't have any choice. I was lying there and I was trembling. Anyway he put a glove on and some KY jelly and he found he couldn't enter me. 'What's the matter with you?' he said and I just burst into tears.

Anyway, he asked me to go back with my husband and he said, 'Did you know your wife suffers from vaginismus?' and my husband said, 'What's that?'. Of course I knew because I'd read about it. I thought, 'Oh God, no,' because I read that these women don't like sex and all that. I was fine with my husband, it was just this doctor.

It happened a couple of times after that and I started to feel somewhat ashamed to have this condition. But it's only been connected with examinations by doctors, never in my private sexual life. I reckon it's to do with having no control or say in the situation. I've no doubt about that at all. It was the same when I was pregnant with my last baby. This doctor wanted to do an internal and I just didn't like him. I said, 'I was promised a woman doctor,' and he said, 'Oh, she can't come over for a routine examination like this,' and I realised then that I was trapped. I was just so tense, I was panicking. The doctor really cursed and swore. He said, 'Oh bloody hell, for Christ's sake can't you relax!' and he just ripped his gloves off and threw them at the bin and walked out. The nurse said, 'You're only trying to get attention, we know all about people like you,' and she went out as well. She couldn't cope with it, I don't think, it was beyond her comprehension. I was in a terrible state. I was absolutally staggered at the way they treated me. That was the last time it happened. I've just not been examined by a male doctor since. I always insist on seeing a woman now.

Many women feel very tense when they are having internal examinations and if you find that you begin to suffer from this kind of panic then it's essential to insist that you see a woman doctor even if it means making an appointment for another day.

If you have a sexual problem it can be very difficult to seek help. Sex-therapy clinics do exist, however, and the Marriage

Guidance Council can very often help. Doctors are not trained to handle anything other than the physical aspects of the problem so whether you choose to discuss it with your GP will depend very much on your relationship with him or her and how much you respect his or her judgement. But with this, as with all health problems, don't just suffer in silence and don't accept all the blame. More often than not sexual problems are the problems of the partnership, not just one of the partners.

Chapter Fourteen

Taking Care

We are our bodies. We owe ourselves respect and not neglect. We should treat ourselves with the same care we lavish on other people. It isn't easy. Often there just doesn't seem to be the time or the money. There are so many pressures to cope with and anyway we've simply got into the habit of putting ourselves second.

We also tend to think of health as the absence of sickness. Provided nothing is actually hurting or itching, we assume that we are fit and well, which is often far from the truth. Most of us don't eat the right food or take enough exercise, in fact we probably recoil from the rather puritanical image of 'sensible' living. When it comes to the pleasures in life, like the song says, 'It's immoral, it's illegal or it makes you fat.' Taking care of ourselves is nothing like as glamorous as that.

I can't pretend that I'm the world's most shining and healthy example of self-care but I'm certainly better than I used to be. I do rest more when under pressure. I do try and eat something nutritious at lunch-time. I do demand time for myself. It takes application. It is, I realise, easier to give advice than it is to take it.

Most of the advice in this chapter I have mentioned elsewhere in the book. It seemed sensible to bring it together again here since this is a dip-into kind of book. Really the basics of good health consist of food, exercise, rest, relaxation and personal hygiene. Other factors such as air pollution and hazards at work are social problems which require political solutions.

Food

One woman told me forcefully during an interview, 'You can't expect your body to work properly if you feed it rubbish.' She was referring to both junk food and all refined and processed foods. People who feel as she does often seem to hold their beliefs with an almost religious fervour which can seem a bit odd and rather off-putting. But we ought to listen because she is correct in her statement, as research has proved. Our diet has an enormous effect on our health because it is food which builds up the body's resistance to disease.

Many of the nutrients in natural food are destroyed by refining and processing. This is why white flour, white sugar and white rice are less useful to the body than brown flour (and bread), brown sugar and brown rice. Tinned and processed foods not only have less nutritional value than natural foods, they have chemicals added as preservatives and colouring which can actually produce an allergic reaction.

It is also known that eating animal fats is associated with heart disease. Milk, butter, cheese, fried foods and fatty meat are all culprits. The lower the level of fat in your diet the better.

Eating wisely really means eating simply. You don't need to be an expert in nutrition. Eat brown and eat fresh and your body will be greatly relieved. Fresh fruit and vegetables are especially healthy and most can be eaten raw or with a minimum of cooking. The real problem is more one of altering our eating and shopping style than of taste or cookery.

We learn patterns of eating as children which can be difficult to un-learn. Most mothers stuff their children with far too much food and take it as a personal rejection if the children don't eat it. Food becomes a major battleground in many families. In fact children will eat a sensible and well-balanced diet if they are left to their own devices. They are much more tuned-in to their body's own needs than adults are. Unfortunately they are rarely left to their own devices and soon fall for the sweet-offerings of a sweet-toothed society. So we grow up eating more than we need of the wrong things and not enough of the right things. It's a bad habit and like all bad habits it takes time and conscious effort to put it right.

Exercise

We are all aware that we should take regular exercise but there are many things which operate against our doing so. For one thing sport is considered a more male activity than a female one. We usually act as the spectators or the people who organise refreshments. It is thought that sport is muscle-building, which isn't considered feminine, but actually strenuous exercise is very healthy and keeps the body fit. It ensures that the blood circulates vigorously and all the body systems are kept from getting sluggish. In the past this was less necessary since women worked so hard on heavy physical labour in the house and in the fields that it happened as a matter of course. Nowadays we have to make an effort, especially if we have a job which keeps us sitting most of the day.

Having young children is one very good way of getting plenty of exercise, of course, as is having an active out-of-doors job. Otherwise we have to look to conventional sports. Swimming is excellent because it exercises all the muscles. It is especially valuable during pregnancy because you can exercise without having to carry all that weight; the water carries it for you.

Jogging is very good, though you have to start slowly and build up your speed and distance as your body get used to the unexpected work. Bicycling can be useful, especially if you can cycle to work every day and so do it regularly. Dance can be very enjoyable in addition to being good exercise, but you have to do it regularly. Team sports can provide a social activity as well as improving your agility and skill. Self-defence sports such as judo, jujitsu and karate are good exercise as well as improving your balance and control. They also give you self-confidence. Many women find that yoga works wonders because it not only provides good exercise but also helps you to relax and revitalise your mind.

Whatever exercise you decide to do, don't rush at it; build it up slowly or you will over-tax your body and feel very stiff and dispirited. Don't eat a big meal before exercise since your body needs energy to digest food and if the energy is being spent elsewhere you are likely to end up with indigestion.

After you have taken exercise give yourself time to calm down and cool down. A hot bath or shower is a useful relaxant and will wash off all the sweat.

Beginning to do strenuous exercise after years of relative idleness can be very discouraging. It's hard work, you're bound to feel stiff and it can easily seem as though the situation will never improve. With effort and patience it will though and you'll feel much better and more in control because of it.

Stress

Stress triggers all kinds of illness. When we are tired and run-down we become more susceptible to infection because the body's natural fighting mechanisms can't operate full blast. Stress occurs as a result of any number of situations. You may have problems at work or problems with your partner. You may have to deal with a family crisis or face unemployment. You may feel depressed or lonely. Dealing with the stress can seem impossible when you are suffering but there are ways of helping yourself.

The first thing is to make sure that you are eating sensibly and regularly. Next, try and do some kind of vigorous exercise, even if it it only bending and stretching. This helps to release tension from your muscles which in turn can ease emotional tension. Mind and body always interact. Deep breathing and relaxation exercises can be equally useful. Some relaxation exercises are described in Chapter 3 (p 34). If you try to practise these regularly they will help to combat the exhaustion which comes with stress.

Dealing with the problems themselves is much more complicated. It's helpful if you are in some sort of crisis to try and do something completely different each day even if it's only going for a long walk, visiting a friend, baking bread, anything you don't normally do as part of the routine of the crisis. Just try to find something that gives you time and space and an activity of your own.

If you are dealing with very painful feelings it can often help to write them down honestly. If you are dealing with a problem which has to be solved, try to see the problem as realistically as possible without getting involved in blaming yourself or someone else for causing it. Whatever the situation, try to avoid putting yourself on a self-improvement course which will make you a 'better' and a 'nicer' person. That always creates stress. We have to learn to accept and like ourselves as we are before it's possible to grow and develop.

Whatever the stress, avoid becoming isolated at all costs. Spend time with friends or members of your family who accept and like you as you are. If you find it difficult to sleep, make time to rest during the day or in the early evening. Many women find yoga or meditation exercises helpful in relieving the pressures. Classes are available in most areas. If you ask at your local library or Citizen's Advice Bureau they should be able to tell you where these are held.

Clothes

Looking after our bodies means making sure they are clean and comfortable. Clothes which are the most fashionable are not always the most healthy. Tight belts, girdles and bras can restrict the circulation. Loose clothing is best. Long skirts can make movement difficult and short skirts make you self-conscious about how you sit and run. High heeled shoes permanently damage the feet and should not be worn all the time.

Many women prefer not to wear bras, finding it more comfortable not to be restricted. Other find it rather painful not to have a bra but need to choose carefully one which isn't too tight. Women who suffer from cystitis and recurrent vaginal infections often choose not to wear pants either. This can be amazingly comfortable but if you don't fancy it, then be sure to buy pure cotton pants which allow your vagina to breathe. Tight trousers, nylon tights and nylon pants are the cause of many vaginal miseries because they retain moisture and provide a good, humid environment in which bacteria can breed.

Personal hygeine

Avoid chemical deodorants, perfumed soaps, bubble bath or introducing any chemical into the water you wash in.

Chemicals can irritate the exquisitively sensitive vaginal skin and cause irritation and inflammation.

The vagina is self-cleaning, a certain amount of discharge is quite normal. It does not need to be scrubbed or perfumed. Douching is not necessary and can be harmful. Research has shown that a high percentage of women who suffer from pelvic infections are habitual and vigorous douchers.

Never put anything in your vagina that you wouldn't put in your mouth.

If for some reason you suffer from a very tender vagina, the most soothing treatment is to add salt to your bath water. This not only soothes, it also cleanses. It also helps if you wash yourself by pouring a jug or bottle of ordinary water at body temperature over the vulva. Facecloths can be abrasive and can also harbour germs.

After going to the toilet, remember to wipe yourself from front to back so that germs from the anus do not reach the urethra or the vagina.

Beware of patent medicines which promise to transform you. One woman I interviewed told me this cautionary tale:

> I was nineteen and I saw this lovely newspaper advertisement that advised me to send away for these pills and within weeks I'd have this marvellous voluptuous bust. So I sent for some and proceeded to take them. There was no visible difference or increase. I was most upset and put it out of my mind. But I stopped menstruating and I got into an awful tizzy, instantly thought I was pregnant, flapped about all over the place, rushed to the boyfriend of the time and said, 'Guess what's happened?' and we got in an awful state. I had groups of friends, all deeply concerned. Then suddenly one of them produced a medical student who started asking all sorts of questions and it just happened to come out that I'd taken these tablets and he said, 'Ah, that's it.' It never occurred to me that that was what caused it. There was nothing on the box. I don't know what they were, some sort of hormone I suppose.

Dealing with doctors

Remember that you can change your doctor, that you can ask for a second opinion and that you do not have to agree to any form of treatment if you do not wish to take it. Our bodies belong to us, we must suffer the consequences of whatever decisions are taken about them. The doctor is simply our technical adviser.

Improving communication with doctors takes time, patience and practise. We see them rarely and they deal with patients every working day. Take a notebook, write down the questions you want to ask and the information you are given. Raise every point that you think might be relevant and explain how you feel if you are anxious. In time your doctor should realise that you are seriously wanting to be involved with your own health care and will co-operate. If s/he consistently puts you down or gets nasty then it's time to change.

Hospital doctors are more difficult to deal with since you rarely see them often enough to form a relationship. But it's important to make up your mind what you will or will not tolerate. If you don't intend to stay in hospital, say so. If you want to be examined by a woman, say so. Don't allow yourself to be pressured to do anything against your better judgement.

We are our bodies. We are our own responsibility. If we take a concerned interest in our health we shall not only feel fitter, we shall feel more confident and in control of our lives.

Further Reading

General medical

Women and Medicine Joyce Leeson & Judith Gray, Tavistock Publications, 1978.

The NHS: Your Money or Your Life Lesley Garner, Pelican Books, 1979.

Complaints and Disorders: the Sexual Politics of Sickness Barbara Ehrenreich and Deirdre English, Writers and Readers Cooperative, 1973.

Health Rights Handbook Gerry and Carol Stimson, Penguin Books, 1978.

Women's health books

Our Bodies Ourselves (British edition) Angela Phillips and Jill Rakusen, Penguin Books, 1978.
The New Women's Health Handbook ed. Nancy MacKeith, Virago, 1978.
My Body My Health Felicia Stewart MD, Felicia Guest, Gary Stewart MD, Robert Hatcher MD, Wiley Medical, 1979 (an American book).
From Woman to Woman Lucienne Lanson, Pelican Books, 1977.
The Fertile Years Wendy Cooper, Arrow Books, 1978.

Specific conditions

Why Suffer? Periods and Their Problems Lynda Birke and Katy Gardner, Virago Handbook, 1979.
Once a Month Katharina Dalton, Fontana, 1978.
The Wise Wound Penelope Shuttle and Peter Redgrove, Penguin Books, 1978.
The Curse Janice Delaney, Mary Jane Lupton, Emily Toth, E.P. Dutton & Co., 1976 (an American book).
Periods Without Pain Erna Wright, Star Books 1966.
No Change Wendy Cooper, Arrow Books, 1976.
Herbs for Female Ailments Sarah Beckett, Thorsons, 1973.
Pre-menstrual Tension June Clark SRN, Hamlyn Paperbacks, 1980.
PMT: the Unrecognised Illness Judy Lever with Dr. M. Brush & Brian Haynes, NEL, 1980.
Understanding Cystitis Angela Kilmartin, Pan Books, 1973.
Cystitis, A Complete Self-Help Guide Angela Kilmartin, Hamlyn, 1980.
Venereal Diseases R. S. Morton, Penguin Books, 1974.
Venereology and Genito-Urinary Medicine R. D. Catterall, Hodder and Stoughton, 1979 (written for nurses but it's readable).
The Life That Lives on Man Michael Andrews, Arrow Books, 1976.
Postnatal Depression Vivienne Welburn, Fontana, 1980.
Not All in the Mind Richard Mackarness, Pan, 1976 (about food allergies).